MW01199424

THE
SCHUBERT
TREATMENT

CLAIRE OPPERT

TRANSLATED BY KATIA GRUBISIC

THE
SCHUBERT
TREATMENT

A STORY OF
MUSIC AND HEALING

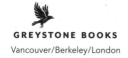

GREYSTONE BOOKS

Vancouver/Berkeley/London

First published in English by Greystone Books in 2024
Originally published in French as *Le Pansement Schubert*,
copyright © 2020 by Éditions Denoël
English translation copyright © 2024 by Katia Grubisic

24 25 26 27 28   5 4 3 2 1

Greystone Books Ltd.
greystonebooks.com

Cataloguing data available from Library and Archives Canada
ISBN 978-1-77840-080-3 (cloth)
ISBN 978-1-77840-081-0 (epub)

Editing for English edition by Paula Ayer
Proofreading by Jennifer Stewart
Jacket and text design by Javana Boothe
Jacket illustration courtesy Library of Congress,
Gertrude Clarke Whittall Foundation Collection, 87752625

Printed and bound in Canada on FSC® certified paper at Friesens. The FSC® label
means that materials used for the product have been responsibly sourced.

Greystone Books thanks the Canada Council for the Arts, the British Columbia
Arts Council, the Province of British Columbia through the Book Publishing Tax
Credit, and the Government of Canada for supporting our publishing activities.

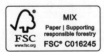

Greystone Books gratefully acknowledges the xʷməθkʷəy̓əm (Musqueam),
Sḵwx̱wú7mesh (Squamish), and səlilwətaɬ (Tsleil-Waututh) peoples on
whose land our Vancouver head office is located.

For my wonderful parents

Contents

Prologue

Schubert, Piano Trio no. 2 in E-flat Major, op. 100
Andante con moto
Exposition

APRIL 2012. PARIS, KORIAN JARDINS D'ALÉSIA.

The leaves of the tall oak quiver in spring's new light in front of the windows of the EHPAD, *the établissement d'hébergement pour personnes âgées dépendantes,* an assisted-living retirement facility.

On the floor for the residents with dementia, the door to the common room we call *l'Espace* is wide open.

Espace—space—is a funny word. The dictionary defines it as the span of the physical universe, the vacuum between the planets, the stars, and the galaxies.

I walk into the common room and turn off the television, just as I do every Monday, a ritual.

The television usually stays on all day long even though no one is watching. When I click it off, the set makes a peculiar noise, like a machine being swallowed, and leaves a flicker of gray in the silence.

The floor for the twenty-one patients with dementia is a closed, protected unit. You need a code for the elevator, which I always forget when I'm standing in front of it. It's funny.

In a corner of the common room, a woman is screaming and struggling. There are two nurses with her, holding her to keep her from sliding down into the chair as they dodge her blows.

The wound on Madame Kessler's* arm is starting to fester, and the nurses have to change the dressing.

I can't see her face, hidden behind the tense, towering nurses, their furrowed brows. She stops screaming just long enough to try to bite them.

I don't know what compels me to go over there. I don't say a word. I sit down and I just play, the andante from Schubert's Piano Trio no. 2 in E-flat Major, op. 100.

Three seconds go by, no time at all, two measures maybe, and her arm relaxes, and drops. The screaming stops. The room goes quiet. Now I can see her face: she looks surprised, and she's almost smiling.

---

*Patient and resident names have been changed to maintain confidentiality.

The nurses are so quick that I don't play for very long. It's more than surprising, it's phenomenal. The nurses smile too. "You'll have to come back," one of them laughs, "for the Schubert treatment."

The phrase is clever, and utterly appropriate. "The Schubert treatment" has been coined, and it will remain.

As I walk away, I already know that something significant has just taken place. For the first time, I have seen evidence of dramatic relief in a person in considerable pain. A year after that spontaneous experiment, when I develop the Schubert treatment protocol, working with over one hundred patients in end-of-life care at the palliative care unit of Sainte-Périne hospital in Paris, the department chief comes up with a pithy, eloquent formula: "Ten minutes of Schubert is the equivalent of five milligrams of oxy."

There will be Schubert, as well as Bach, Mozart, Beethoven, Brahms, Rachmaninoff, Shostakovich, bits of Puccini and Verdi, Édith Piaf, crooners like Claude François, Michel Sardou, Salvatore Adamo, even some Johnny Hallyday, waltzes and tangos, Jewish, Arab, and African music, folk songs from Brittany and Ireland, movie soundtracks, jazz, rock and roll, pop, heavy metal...

That same week, I come back twice to play for Madame Kessler as the nurses change her dressing, with the same results. There's no other way to alleviate her pain. She sits in her chair, ramrod straight, holding her arm out for the nurses, and as I play the andante from Schubert's Trio over and over again her face glows, so intensely luminous that it lights up the whole room, the nurses, and me. Outside, the wide branches of the oak are bathed in light. At least, that's how it looks to me when I bid the tree farewell.

A Good Story

I will strive to cleave as closely as possible to the events of the past twenty-five years, and to trace the mysterious ways music works when it truly moves patients: those referred to as deeply autistic, care-home residents, dementia patients, people with painful illnesses, and those who are at the end of their lives.

My story isn't logical; rather, it bears witness to that sovereign, virgin heart, the true core of us that music can sometimes reach and revive.

It's a good story, a happy story.

What pushed the musician I was toward a care profession wasn't a moral imperative but something natural, instinctive; something innate.

Music, in the curved form of the cello, became my life, and stood like a bulwark against absurdity, disease, and death, to try to reach the thing that lies beneath, the thing that resists. Subterranean. Bedside music. Trust: a refreshing wind.

The recognition of life's fragile grace.

Gratitude that flows like so many streams.

Paul

Bach, Cello Suite no. 1 in G Major, prelude
Slow, joyful

MARCH 1997. SAINT-DENIS, ADAM SHELTON CENTER, medical and educational institute for children and young people with autism.

His nose pressed up against the window that separates the hallway from the room I'm in, Howard watches me play the cello, like every Friday. I play in front of Paul; I am playing for Paul.

Paul is fifteen years old. He has autism. He's a stunning child, with an unexpected kind of beauty, and intense blue eyes. Paul has never spoken. He's sitting cross-legged, facing the wall, rocking back and forth fitfully, his back stiff, his eyes staring at some faraway point. Now and again he tips his head back, laughs loudly, and stops. His face is contorted by anxiety. Paul spits, he pisses on the floor in front of me, he laughs again, even louder. Sometimes his gaze runs through me, but he doesn't really see me. It's so strange.

As he rocks, he makes a noise, a continuous hum, like an engine, with a few gruff syllables. It's hard to describe, halfway between laughing and sobbing.

From the back of the room, I start to hum, to moan, and to rock just like him. It's the only thing I can think of doing in that moment. My cello hasn't started to sing yet, but I can feel the ancient wood pressed against my chest; it's part of my body. Paul comes closer, shuffling over on his bum. He's so close, and suddenly he spits up into the air with surprising precision. He gathers the spittle in his hands and spreads it carefully all over his face. For a second, his wet fingers brush against my cello. He sniffs the instrument's fingerboard. He wants me to sniff too. He's whining impatiently, and he starts rocking faster, inches away from me, clutching my hair. It's as if it's not me at all, as if I'm not even here. I don't struggle, and I don't say anything. At last, he lets go. He holds his head in his hands and smacks his cheeks, hard, one after the other. As if it's not him. As if he's not even here. He's crying.

I start to play the prelude to Bach's First Cello Suite. As soon as the first notes ring out, Paul goes still and stops crying. He jumps to his feet. He runs to get a long plastic tube from the corner of the room and brings it up to his eyes, pointing it in my direction. It seems like he's finally seeing me. That's the impression I get. Or maybe he's looking at the music flowing toward him, within him. I don't know. I didn't even know these questions existed.

What I do know is that I'm not afraid, I feel good with him. And he feels good with me.

A cloud of breath has formed on the other side of the glass, like when children play against a window. A squashed, twisted nose. Howard's eyes are full of tears.

What does he see that I don't? Howard Buten is a clinical psychologist, an expert in extreme cases, the direst cases that all the other institutions have turned away.

> *They obviously have so much to teach us, even when*
> *what they do frightens us.*
>
> HOWARD BUTEN

Paul is smiling, a luminous shadow subtly gleaming beneath his stormy brow and blue eyes. He puts down the plastic tube and comes to sit near me again. He is calm. He lays his right cheek and his two hands flat on the top of the cello. I think he's singing.

Through the Wall

I'm very young. I'm a little girl, we're in my family's apartment in Paris, and before I fall asleep I call to my mother through the bedroom wall: "Maman! I'm happy!" I say it over and over.

I feel light; there is something clear and bright riveted to my heart.

Happiness courses through the wall that separates my bedroom and that of my beloved mother.

The feeling has never changed. I still feel that same sense of wonder.

A sparkle from the wellspring of days.

Trust and gratitude before the splendor of all things: this is life's foundation, its bedrock.

Paul, the Explosion

Bach, Cello Suite no. 5 in C Minor, prelude
Somber

THERE IS A HORRIBLE BANG, like the blast of a cannon, war, the echo in the trenches. The cello has split. The top of the instrument is broken. Paul punched his fist right through the wood. Never in my life, not even in my worst nightmares, have I ever imagined a cello breaking like that, right against my chest. The sensation is indescribable, the violence unthinkable. I freeze, my heart pounding, stunned by what has just happened.

"Paul, Paul, what have you done? Paul, Paul…"

A shiver runs through my body. My heart is ravaged. I feel very alone all of a sudden.

The cello is broken, gaping, yet after the initial shock, I accept it.

"It's okay, Paul. I'll keep playing."

I can still play. The body is splintered along the left side, but the bridge and the strings haven't moved, and the cello is even still in tune.

I'm shaking a little, and I change what I was playing. I start Edvard Grieg's "Solveig's Song."

During our next sessions, Paul sits cross-legged and trails his hand in the gap, in the hollow of the splintered cello. It's a caress that might turn dangerous, sensuous, repeated over and over.

From time to time, he casts me a sidelong glance.

After that incident, Howard forbids me from reading anything on autism. He makes me swear that I won't do any research. "Swear, you have to swear. Right here, right now." I swear, my heart beating fast.

"It's amazing what you're doing with them, with the cello."

In the six years I spend working with Howard and his family of autistic kids, I never once so much as look at a book or read an article about autism.

One day, in the summer, exactly four months after my first session with Paul, I risk Bach's Fifth Cello Suite again. I haven't dared play it since his last outburst—out of instinct, out of fear, both for me and for him. And what happens still astounds me today.

After three measures, again, he punches the instrument. The hole in the top is gaping wide, but the strings are still hanging on. A sliver of wood hangs on under the bridge.

The cello is fatally wounded.

For the first time, Paul looks right at me. Neither one of us moves. He is sounding the depths of me, endlessly, fascinated. Our eyes meet, the gaze permeating everything.

> *You have to look at them straight in the eye, and you*
> *have to be so welcoming, so open, so guileless and*
> *without judgment that they can't resist.*
>
> H.B.

Paul never hit the cello again. I never again played the prelude to Bach's Fifth Cello Suite. And we spent several more years together. During every session, he always looked at me straight on, and always his wet fingers wandered with such delight, exploring the open belly of the cello.

Yes, Howard, there is someone in there, without a doubt.

Howard

1974, United States. Detroit, the Children's Orthogenic Center.

Howard Buten was twenty-four when he met Adam Shelton, a child with autism.

He describes Adam as a hurricane wrapped up in a boy's skin, who tumbled into his waiting room and threw himself on the floor, his legs stiff, rocking back and forth, staring into space, "his hoarse voice spitting out syllables as if he'd swallowed something, but hadn't." So Howard threw himself on the floor too, like Adam, maybe because, as he says, he wanted to show his admiration for the boy.

During the years that followed, Howard devoted himself entirely to Adam. And since that day, he has been obsessed with one question: Why does he feel so at home around patients with autism?

"Home," he emphasizes; "Where the heart is."

Howard was born in Detroit. From a very young age, he played violin, sang, danced. He was a mime, a magician, a ventriloquist;

he dreamed of running away to join the circus. His mother, herself a former child performer who used to say that she'd retired at sixteen, taught Howard tap dancing and figure skating. He was an acrobat, he learned to juggle and ride a unicycle. He tried the trumpet, the drums, guitar, percussion, and finally composition.

A year before he met Adam, Howard created a clown character, Buffo.

He's also a doctor of clinical psychology, who came to some renown in France after the success there of his book When I Was Five I Killed Myself.

One day, Howard told me that if someone held a gun to his head and forced him to choose between his three professions—clown, psychologist, writer—he would choose his autistic family.

He was standing in front of me among the kids, his index finger against his temple, not moving, not smiling, glancing all around.

Amélia

Bach, Cello Suite no. 2 in D Minor, prelude
Soft, tender

Amélia bangs her head. Backward, forward. She bites. She pinches and scratches. If she doesn't draw blood, she comes back and scratches again. She is extremely aggressive with others—the other kids at the center, the patient-care attendants, her family. And with the other within her as well.

Today, my hands are scarred after my session with her. Blood as the ultimate form of communication. Amélia has just turned eighteen.

As she listens to the cello, she howls like a wolf. She only likes soft music. The slow movement of Schubert's Arpeggione Sonata gradually calms her down.

She arrived at the center about a year after me. Until then, she had been in a psychiatric institution, in restraints for two years and completely knocked out by powerful antipsychotics for the last few months. Howard told us how he got her out of the hospital, a Byzantine undertaking. Howard never abandons a patient. Once, while Buffo was touring in the Czech Republic, he flew to Paris and back in a single day to make sure Paul got his meds.

On the morning she arrived, Amélia was released into the center. That's Howard's word, *released*. I wasn't there that day, but when I came back I found out she had gone on a rampage with a fire extinguisher she ripped out of the wall. The Adam Shelton Center had to be closed for two days for repairs.

> *Some days, I tell myself that in the end I'm going to*
> *buy myself a desert island, and I'm going to go get*
> *every person with autism on earth and take them*
> *all with me.*

H.B.

Howard dreams of creating a world in which Amélia's violence is not experienced as violence, and therefore doesn't exist.

How many times have I seen him come back from the room in the basement, his face scratched, torn up, blood trickling down his forehead after sessions with particularly violent kids, the ones he calls his hard cases, like Djamel. Djamel has only one goal—ripping out everybody's eyes. He favors underhanded, surprise attacks. Djamel is dangerous. Howard, in his basement universe, does his best to dance around, to avoid Djamel's teeth, nails, and fists, without fear, or at least without showing him any fear. In that world, Howard accepts the bites, scratches, and blows he can't avoid. The rest of the time, he mimics the children. He's not going to cure them, obviously. He transforms them.

Music makes Amélia want to come closer to me. Is it just the music? She's out for blood, and then she's all sweetness and caresses, her gestures imbued with an unfamiliar tenderness when she comes near the cello. There is a furtive smile in the darkness of her apparent absence from the world. As she listens to the music, her eyes sparkle so brightly that I worry she's going to start a fire.

Two years after her arrival here, Amélia is a different person.

On the center's bulletin board, Howard puts up a picture of Amélia her mother sent in: Amélia sitting next to the Christmas tree, surrounded by the whole family, smiling.

My Father

I might have become a doctor, like my brother, like my father, like my grandfather. That was my dream.

My father was a doctor and an artist.

He was late sometimes when he called on his patients—five hours, seven hours, two days. His relationship with time was idiosyncratic, to put it mildly.

"The doctor was always late, never absent."

At midnight he would ring the doorbell, walk into the apartment, and ask for soup, because he hadn't had supper. Later, he sat down at the piano, played one of Chopin's nocturnes, often no. 20 in E-flat major, then he closed the fallboard, put on a hat that was always too small, and took his leave. Doctor, the patient might say, you didn't examine me. *To which he replied, quite matter-of-factly,* Everything is much better, I'll see you next week.

"The doctor often sat at the piano, since music is a call to life."

My father was a baffling man, and an artist.

He traveled all over France and beyond to visit his patients.

Everywhere he was welcomed, and loved. He didn't always take money but would gladly accept homemade rhubarb compote, Caribbean rice pudding, or fresh vegetable soup.

"The indefatigable doctor, attentive beyond all reason, the doctor whose intuition was akin to genius, whose diagnosis never erred, whose ethics were impeccable, and whose selflessness was authentic because it was natural."

He was the company doctor for several theaters in Paris, including the Odéon and the Madeleine, and he often brought me to the shows. We were always late: I think I never saw the first act of a play. We would barge into the theater and disturb a whole row. Pardon me, excuse me. *People had to get up to let us go by. Later, during my own concerts, from the stage, as I watched the lights dim in the theater, his seat would still be empty, then, suddenly, in the middle of the movement of a sonata, the row would rise a bit at a time and his bowed form carve itself out of the darkness.* Pardon me, excuse me. *He sidled to his seat, sending out slight, carefree ripples through the audience. He had not an ounce of shame. During intermission, he went up to strangers at random—*Did you like it?*—and without waiting for an answer, he announced with childlike pride,* Did you know that's my daughter? Yes, yes! That's my daughter.

"The doctor always devoted, never overbearing, always completely present, never aloof."

My father was utterly unique.

He was a man who defied labels, the kind of man who split everything in two in order not to have to choose one person over another. He always shared his bread, regardless of how much he had, his soup, he shared the medication that filled his pockets. Shortly before he died, of mandibular cancer, he was sharing his morphine.

"The consummate doctor, an artist of what it is to be human."

My father, the enigma.

Dîlan

Bach, Cello Suite no. 3 in C Major, prelude
Joyful, with gratitude

Every Friday, before I push open the large glass doors and walk into the center, I can already hear the screams in the garden. My presence has been noted. How does Dîlan know I'm here before I've even arrived? No one at the center has ever been able to answer that question. She claps her hands and screeches with delight as she skips around in that twitchy way she has. "Here comes Claire," one of the teachers says.

Dîlan is Kurdish. She's fourteen years old. She has green eyes and light hair. Her hoarse voice modulates up to long, high-pitched squeals and down to probing lows. She rushes frenetically into the room set aside for our cello session.

When I settle in to play, she gets even more excited. She comes up to me and takes my hands, places them on the fingerboard and drags them up and down the strings. That means, *Play me the harmonics in the allegro from Shostakovich's Sonata.* Dîlan is a fine musician, with very specific tastes. Above all she loves the explosive, repetitive, sarcastic movement in the Sonata that I've been playing for weeks. And if I should chance other repertoire, she goes crazy and jumps on me to put my left hand back on the fingerboard and show me the movement up and down the strings: the allegro from Shostakovich's Sonata. She knows exactly what she wants, and she knows how to ask for it. Like Paul, Dîlan has never spoken a word in her life.

Music seems to make up for the absence of language. In the very depths of her being, she has some form of musical prescience, the evidence of which can be seen in her frantic wincing as she listens to every inflection in the melody—she's tense when the cello sings the first development, there's the ecstasy of the recapitulation, and she relaxes with the ebb back to the original key. She listens to the cello in a state of paroxysmal joy. She tosses her head and howls with pleasure. She always leans against the radiator. Her head bangs ferociously against the wall. Once, she slipped down to the floor and bashed her head against the radiator, bleeding profusely. She doesn't feel pain. She kept laughing and clapping her hands. She wiped the blood and, her cheeks aflame, asked again for the Shostakovich allegro.

So much has been written about autism. As Howard often says, the more you read, the more you get lost in it, and the more you write about what little we do know, the more rampant the mystery and contradictions. Every time anyone says, *autism is...*, there will always be a case when it is not.

I give in and pick up some information here and there, innocently, despite my original promise. I learn that some people think there's a biological cause, while others think it's psychological, and still others believe the cause of autism is genetic. I find out that the early descriptions of pediatric autism include linguistic anomalies and a "powerful desire for aloneness and sameness." I read lists of clinical criteria: communication difficulties, withdrawal, stereotyped gestures, a resistance to environmental change, a lack of emotional affect.

Howard says he's never met a single person with autism who wasn't good company or with whom he wasn't able to communicate. It's less obvious from the outside, he explains, though he can feel it every time. My cello and I feel it too, every time.

> *I believe they should be loved for what they are and not for what they ought to be or what they should become.*
>
> H.B.

Music touches the child through what Howard calls their "invisible wall," into unsuspected depths.

Where words are inaccessible, sometimes music—its silent breath—can reach below ground.

A sense of trust.

The purveyance of joy.

The Cello

I'm six years old. My first piano teacher is a charming lady with gray hair pulled back in a bun, and a wrinkled face. My most vivid memory of her is the giant Melba toasts slathered in strawberry jam she fed me before every lesson.

I'm eight, and my parents take me into Paris one afternoon to hear a concert by one of their friends, a talented pianist, an older man who has all but retired from the stage. He's playing the Beethoven sonatas with a young cellist.

It's love at first sight: I fall for the instrument as violently and suddenly as a lightning strike.

The cello sings with its warm, round, plaintive voice. From the first sound, I recognize my forever instrument.

On our way home, I announce to my parents, "I want to play the cello."

I'm fourteen and playing my first concert at the Noailles hotel in Saint-Germain-en-Laye. I'm playing a Giuseppe Sammartini sonata for cello and piano. I have a lump in my throat and I'm trying not to cry because I played a wrong note near the end of the last movement.

A woman comes to stand before me at the end of the concert. I don't remember her face, but I can still see how pale she was, her headwrap, and the light in her eyes.

"If you were a doctor, you would have healed me."

What I especially remember is the shock wave her words sent through me.

The fierce recognition of a founding intuition.

An immersive wave cresting slowly in the bottom of my soul.

David

Bach, Cello Suite no. 4 in E-flat Major, prelude
Sorrowful

JANUARY 2001. SAINT-DENIS, ADAM SHELTON CENTER.

David weighs two hundred and forty pounds. Two teachers drag him into the room where I'm waiting to see him. He's always getting dragged somewhere by someone, his usual means of locomotion. They place him in a corner of the room, knees up, arms wrapped tight, his ungainly body curled up on itself, folded into as many segments as possible. His head is hunched into his neck, and he is facing the wall, his fingers digging into his eyes. David is eighteen years old. He's neither deaf nor mute, but he too is nonverbal. He doesn't respond to his name.

He lies down on the floor, his face still turned toward the wall. Silence. When I start playing the cello, he hunches over even more, gathering the whole unwieldy mass of his body. He presses his fingers deeply into his eyes and places his thumbs over his ears. Next to his ears, actually: his ears aren't really even shaped like ears, just tiny holes on either side of his face. They're nearly invisible; I almost wonder whether, after years of silence, they've lost their shape and gone smooth. All it takes is a slight pressure to block out all the noise. Silence.

I play for David every Friday for a year, all of Bach's suites, into the silence of those ears closed up tight. He's heard all six cello suites in their entirety several times. Nine times: Howard counted one Friday afternoon, calculating it all very seriously.

> *First, you have to earn their attention. It's up to*
> *us to find a way to be interesting to their eyes… to*
> *change and to reinvent every time.*
>
> H.B.

After three weeks, David takes his hands away from his ears and risks a glance in my direction. Quickly, he plugs his ears again.

In early spring, David smiles. For the first time, then a second time. It's a smile full of light, a miraculous smile.

He smiles more often and for longer when the cello is singing. One day, he turns around abruptly, flipping his entire body toward me with a dull thud. Sometimes he reminds me of a gigantic fish.

He no longer covers his ears. He listens. Finally, at the beginning of May, he drags himself over to my cello. He touches it, smells it for a long time, licks it. He lays his head on the top of the instrument. He looks truly happy.

In June, when David sits up and climbs up on the stool in front of the piano by himself, Howard, fascinated, joins us and sits down quietly.

David has never learned to play piano. He doesn't know how to play. And yet we begin our first musical conversations. The trust is absolute; the risk, too. Until that moment, I have never known the joy of this kind of conversation. I feel like I've never been privy to any musical exchange as deep as this one.

Some things are enough to justify an entire lifetime, and David slowly sitting up, over the time it takes me to play all of the Bach cello suites through nine times, is without a doubt one of them.

David lives in a world of disharmonious musical intervals. On the keyboard, he plays exclusively minor sevenths, a tense, unstable interval, in a nervous, syncopated rhythm, over and over again, with one finger of each hand. A-flat/G-flat, A-flat/G-flat... Howard has dubbed this new piano technique the "two-finger method."

For months, we play back and forth. David has started following my directions—David, who never even responds to his own name. "It's my turn, David." He lets me play, stooped over the stool, half smiling, waiting for me to finish. "It's your turn, David."

I believe they have to be educated, they have to prac-
tice communicating, regardless of the result.

H.B.

Although he never moves beyond his two-finger technique, his playing evolves considerably. At first, he just looks
at the white keys without venturing to touch them, barely
stroking those two soft flats. One day, he crosses the threshold and dares to touch the white keys, striking a more candid
sound. Then he finds his favorite interval an octave below and
stays there for a long time, reveling in the sound of the same
thing played differently. He has only ever played it broken,
and now for the first time he plays both notes of the interval,
hitting those two familiar notes in a new way. He stops for
a moment. He looks perplexed. He reacts the same way the
day he discovers that he can slow the tempo down by exactly
half. His musical experiments play out at the boundary of
the known and unknown. He laughs a lot, and I find I do too.
He's diversifying his relationship to sound. He's exploring. I
answer with my instrument. I copy him, step by step, I imitate
everything he does. Little by little, although he maintains the
structure of his interval, he expands his auditory range and

reaches toward lower and higher sounds on the keyboard. I try the same thing on the cello. I watch him displace his torso toward the right side of the keyboard, although he remains glued to the seat, stretching his arms and neck to reach the highest notes. Sometimes he gets stuck up there, and I have to get up and use all my strength to set him upright again. He always waits for new instructions to continue his explorations. Then he heads off in the other direction, going left, down the keyboard. After a few weeks, he starts moving his stool himself. He laughs and laughs, joyful in the uninterrupted give-and-take of our two voices, and in the compliance too.

Your gaze has to become a house, built expressly for them, the door wide open, painted in their colors and furnished to their taste.

H.B.

I drag David along. Since he stopped covering his ears, he can't resist. The cello sings with its warm, round, plaintive voice, and it takes hold of his body. He's drawn by the vibration. The repertoire doesn't matter to him. I head out toward unknown lands, on pure intuition, spinning far beyond the limits of anything that I know, of what I've learned. My improvisations push the limits of the instrument too. After alternating, our voices merge, his voice and mine combined.

Now I say it like an order: "Together, David." The strings of my instrument cry out beneath the impatient bow. The tempo picks up, melodies unravel. He reacts immediately. The sound of the cello gushes into the secret breaches in the invisible wall of David's self, and now and again makes it through. Swells, scratches, squeaks, moans, whimpers, whistles, sobs, pleas, hiccups, gasps, quiet. Silence, sometimes.

Our playing is a call and answer, our voices interwoven. We learn crescendo, from pianissimo to fortissimo. David follows along with me, docile. He hits the keys of the piano harder and harder every time. He loves it. When I start the dramatic decrescendo, sometimes he refuses to follow. Usually, I manage to keep him with me, to bring him back on the path toward peace, toward a silence woven through with echoes.

> *Since no one really knows what to do [for autistic patients], the only choice we have is unconditional respect.*
>
> H.B.

Sometimes I invite myself over to his disharmonious universe, and then he's the one who drags me along, into the void. David's world is a world in motion. I step over the border, sinking dangerously. These ways are new to me, I can feel that. They're new to him too as he moves toward me. The beat of him and the beat of me are so perfectly in sync that we can't always tell the timbre of the two instruments apart. We fall into each other. It's incredible.

If I leave suddenly, if I veer off without warning in a different musical direction, toward my own territory, made of more so-called harmonious intervals, more stable intervals, or toward an unexpected, sketched-out attempt at some tune, it's like I'm trying to force him to meet me on my shore. Am I pushing him? Betraying him? Right away, he rips his fingers off the keyboard as if he's been burned, and he tries to cover his ear holes again, stunned. The border crossing between the discordant and the consonant. David isn't completely docile after all. He can withdraw, too.

> *I want to know what in the world it could possibly feel like to be him.*
>
> H.B

Does music allow David to express himself? Does it evoke new sensations and emotions? Is he really creating a sound universe that is his own?

"A storyless journey through the hilly, heady land of pure emotional sensation": that's how Howard describes our musical excursions.

I don't know how I manage to guess what piece to play and how to play it for these supposedly noncommunicative children. I know which Bach suite calms Paul down or turns him into a cello killer; I know the tune that settles Amélia enough for her to stop tearing at my hands, for her scratches to become kisses; I know which sonata movement makes Dîlan almost levitate with joy; and I know the musical interval that has the power to stand David up and allow him to become, on occasion, a concert pianist.

What I don't know yet, since I've read nothing, or almost nothing, is that instinctively, I'm using the same methods Howard has used and fine-tuned his whole life—imitation and empathy.

Encounter

1996. Paris, the Louvre auditorium.

The first time I met Howard Buten was during a colloquium on art and medicine, an event I happened upon somewhat by accident. I say met, but it wasn't quite a meeting.

I heard him speak to a packed room, and I couldn't manage to get close to him at the end of the lecture. Howard Buten is a man who gets lots of media attention, and that night, the lineup was long.

The only sentence I remember from his talk is his laconic answer to a fluttering lady in the audience, with his now-familiar American accent: "L'autisme? On n'en sait rien." We know nothing.

In the awkward silence that followed his declaration—a surprising statement by an internationally renowned clinical specialist on autism—something started shaking inside me, a strange resonance that stirred up the same powerful joy I felt as a child when that woman with cancer spoke to me after my first concert.

A few weeks after that, I went to see Buffo the clown at the Ranelagh in Paris.

Buffo comes forward on the stage, his face chalky, his eyes darkened with kohl. He wonders aloud about the world around him, finding few answers. Buffo has plenty of troubles, but he usually muddles through; he has lots of disappointment, but happy moments too. A character of pure poetry, deeply melancholy, never sentimental.

He pops out of the darkened wings in his enormous shoes, and holding a rubber chicken. There is a cello, too, and Buffo is clearly enamored of the instrument. The cello is caught in a spotlight that shines onto the stage, and at the back of its wooden body is a little door. Every night, Buffo delicately opens the door and extracts a tiny violin, rocking it tenderly against his heart for a long time.

How brave, or, rather, how brazen of me to barge into his dressing room. An undertow of confidence binds me to myself.

The presumption of kinship.

Again, I feel that wave unfurl from the bottom of my heart. One day, when I know him better, Howard will talk about the same feeling, which grabs him the same way and has since he was very young, whenever he encounters certain things or certain people: "It's a feeling you can't name, you can't describe it. It's neither sadness nor joy. But it's strong. It's pure emotion."

"Hello, I'm a cellist. Can we work together?"

I will come to learn that Howard is not afraid of silence. He looks at me for a long time, a very long time, with his wide, sad, smile-creased eyes.

His answer is brief: "I'll be in touch."

Holding Space

Saint-Saëns, "The Swan"

MAY 2012. PARIS, KORIAN JARDINS D'ALÉSIA.

The leaves of the tall oak in front of the windows sway gracefully in their green dress, waiting for summer.

It's nap time, and most of the residents are sleeping in chairs. I turn off the television and say hello to Madame Olivier, who is dozing at the round table, her eyelids flickering behind her thick glasses. She's a massive woman, with swollen, twisted feet, who can only be moved around with a hoist. She's been diagnosed with schizophrenia. Every Monday, when she wakes up, she looks at me with palpable anguish. Nothing about her attitude hints at the miracle to come.

The residents start drifting into the room, into l'Espace, like a disorganized army. Some shuffle in with a cane, others with a walker. Others still are wheeled in slowly by attendants. The patients who are already in the room are brought closer to the round table, which is piled with percussion instruments, maracas, rainsticks, and bells, as well as scarves, paint, leaves, flowers, and branches.

Some come in screaming, shattering the silence with insults. Others are mute. One woman rushes in, deftly deking all the obstacles in her way. She sits down very quickly, stands back up and sits down again, makes as if to leave, and sits down once more. She's been doing this all day, every day, for three years, with unstoppable energy. No one pays any attention to her.

Madame Beaurivage wheels in, like royalty, her hair impeccably done, wearing a flowered blouse and a gold pendant, her face locked up tight. When the attendant wheels her to her spot, she starts yelling at her violently: "You idiot! Get out, you bitch!" She looks around at the other residents condescendingly: "What the hell am I doing here?" Without waiting for an answer, she goes on, "I wanted to be a singer, but my parents said, you have a voice, so you'll be a lawyer." She says the same thing at the start of each one of our one hundred and twenty-two sessions together. After turning off the television set, another ritual, the unchanging prelude to her impressive interpretations of Schubert's lieder and of French songs. It's true, she does have a splendid voice, powerful and velvety, a real opera voice.

I sit down cheerfully in the circle, among these people, all of whom are broken in some way. The cello sings. Saint-Saëns's swan alights in the middle of the table.

To my left, Madame Kessler smiles at the music and moans impatiently.

"Oh, my dear... You're finally here!"

Madame Tisserand, Madame Barthélemy, Madame Joly, Madame Renard, and Monsieur Lemaître sit around the table, joining our group. Madame Tisserand goes fluttery at the sound of the cello, and Madame Beaurivage barks at her.

"Shut up! Will you shut up?!"

"You! You be quiet!" Madame Kessler breaks in. "You're wrecking the music!"

"Shut up!" Madame Beaurivage shouts again, glancing around, half furious, half amused.

Next to them, her hands delicately placed on her knees, her face radiant, Madame Barthélemy is already humming, eyes cast up to the ceiling. She has stopped her usual impenetrable logorrhea. Madame Joly sits back with her eyes closed and her head reclining, drooling profusely. A slight smile slices the parchment of her face in two. As for Monsieur Lemaître, he says nothing at all, curled up, his face tucked in his elbow, smiling within himself.

Saint-Saëns's "The Swan" takes flight, opening its wings wide over the cluttered table, brushing against the bells and the leaves. Shyly, with ancient hands, they try to grab the swan's wings, and, in an exquisite murmur, the dance is born. The air goes white with sound and voices. The whole room, all the space in l'Espace lifts as the metamorphosis begins. Something quakes and the bodies take flight, every heart held aloft in the amber light.

The attendants, who until then have been standing back, like they're part of the furniture, start to move too. First they smile, and clap their hands. They dance, they even waltz. For forty-five minutes, one hundred and twenty-two times over five years, invariably, shouting gives away to shared song.

A sense of trust.

The purveyance of joy.

When the swan flies up to the blue sky, Madame Tisserand starts humming again softly, sneaking a glance at Madame Beaurivage. But Madame Beaurivage is already singing, and her voice is sublime. With his head peeking out of his elbow, Monsieur Lemaître is tapping his fingers slowly against the table. Madame Joly looks at me through barely open eyes, and her emaciated feet are moving imperceptibly to the music. In her otherwise immobile body, the tiny movements of her toes are bigger than even the widest wings opened up to the sun.

Madame Kessler sings and looks at me, her eyes shining. She grabs the drum in front of her and beats along, euphoric.

When the swan leaves the room and disappears over the horizon as the cello sighs that last, long note, the room is filled with a suspended, violet springtime stillness: "The swans take flight…" I speak first, the first line of the poem, to invite the words of others. Madame Kessler picks up the invisible thread of a poem being born.

Her voice surges forth like an invocation:

The dynasty of swans taking flight.
Oh, white swan…
I see you red against the blue sky.

It's like a wind gusting through: through her voice, some spirit refreshes our cracked-open hearts—a light breeze, a calamitous hurricane. New words spring up, the clamor of the drum, bells pealing. An extraordinary feeling takes hold of us and swoops us up. I play the birth of the swan and the flight once more, I play its death and resurrection, and the soft melody mixes with the rustle of wings gone blood red. Words tumble out and jumble together from the belly of sounds, mad vowels tossed out haphazardly, stuttering consonants, grandiose prose.

"The swan is coming," Madame Kessler declares, "it's opening its wings."

"Its wings," Madame Tisserand says again; she's aphasic and repeats in echolalia, catching her fellow residents' words mid-flight like specks of dust floating in a beam of light. "Wings, wings…"

"The swan is embodied grace," Madame Kessler adds, "the beauty of everything that is untainted."

"Its wings," Madame Tisserand insists, "its wings."

Madame Renard tiptoes into the poem, whispering, "Without intercession."

And Madame Olivier shouts, "Straight to the heart!"

"To the heart," Madame Tisserand reiterates, "to the heart."

Madame Olivier is watching me out of the corner of her eye, terrified of saying or doing the wrong thing.

"It's beautiful," Madame Beaurivage sings, since she only ever says anything by singing it.

"It's beautiful," Madame Olivier repeats, "my God, it's beautiful."

"My God, my God…"

The words bounce around faster and faster and my cello is already singing a new song, a languid serenade, a minuet, a light waltz, a tango, a melancholy elegy, or a love song, to accompany the poem being created, to midwife it into being and continue the journey. The song begets the poem. And the poem bursts out of every throat, transforming the dementia circle into a room full of troubadours, minstrels, cantors.

All of those who can't speak or sing are waving colorful scarves with trembling hands, rattling bells and percussion instruments. Without even thinking about it, the attendants join in. The silk scarves soar into the air like bright arabesques, undulating with the melody, tangling and untangling over the wheelchairs. Around the table people are dancing in a hundred different ways, with their feet, their hands, their chins, sometimes just with their eyes. Sometimes a blink is enough to join the dance.

And the gesture born of the strength of sound makes silent speech visible, deployed across the room, across the space—interstellar, intergalactic.

The silk-winged swan has become joy.

Russia

October 1989. Moscow.

The Belorusskiy train station is crowded and bustling on this frozen morning. A fifty-hour train ride. I've crossed both Germanies, Poland, Byelorussia, Ukraine, and part of Russia, its endless snowy plains, with my nose against the window and my cello always by my side.

The vodka-tipsy conductor helps me carry off two metal trunks filled with everything that's supposed to be lacking in Soviet Russia. I hardly speak the language. My heart is full to bursting. My Russian dream is about to come true and nothing else seems important to me right now. I'm going to be studying cello at the Moscow Conservatory.

I don't yet know that these four years will change my life forever.

The student center at the conservatory is a long brick building, beyond dilapidated. I'll be sharing a small room with an Armenian violinist from Baku. Shortly after I arrive, her entire family moves in, fleeing Azerbaijan.

We sleep with our coats on because several of the window panes are broken, and in spite of the bundles of cotton we try to stuff in the gaps between the double windows, the Russian winter's cold is biting.

We shower wearing high-heeled plastic shoes: the communal stalls are so filthy that no one wants to venture in barefoot. Half the time, the showerhead is missing, stolen by the previous occupant. I end up getting my own and I bring it with me every time I shower, screw it in, and then take it back to my room for the next time.

At the conservatory, the most basic processes become complex undertakings. Every morning, before the sun peeks over the horizon, I hop out of my frozen bed to reserve a room in the basement with Panya, the keeper of the repetitoriy, the rehearsal rooms. She's a squat babushka with a large face out of a Russian folktale and a flowered kerchief on her head. She spends all day crossing herself. She calls me by sweet little nicknames and hugs me tight every time she sees me. In the halls, I cross paths with a few lost rats and dazed students, looking troubled, staggering about as they search in vain for the way back to their rooms.

Working with my own cello spares me the pianists' daily disappointments. They play on broken instruments, with missing keys, the pedals long lost or stolen. I don't know how many times I've seen a student walking around in the basement halls with a whole piano keyboard under their arm, or hauling down a repetitoriy door to replace one that inexplicably vanished during the night.

A friend of mine, a French violinist, hates how dirty it is, and every day he takes a taxi to the French embassy to use their bathroom.

We eat badly, with little variety. After I run out of what I brought from France, I start looking out for produkty—*food—in the lineups that form in the middle of the street or in front of stores. You grab a spot and start asking the same question over and over again: What's for sale? With any luck, a few bananas, or, miraculously, sometimes even a few pounds of bananas. I slide into the long lineup I can't even see the end of, hoping to find something good to eat, and I ask the person ahead of me what they're selling. Vacuum cleaners, comes the indifferent answer, and as I wander away, I hear furious, indignant voices cry, "Hey! Don't give out more than five at a time!"*

The waiting is interminable, and it's a part of daily life here. When I want to try to call my parents in France, I take a taxi to the zentralny telegraf, *the central post office, which is an hour away from the student center. After several hours, my number is finally called and it's my turn to use the wooden phone booth. If there's no one home, which is usually the case, well, too bad, and I just head back, having wasted all that time for nothing. I hail a pirate taxi and negotiate the few rubles' ride back across the tentacular city of Moscow.*

Sometimes the cars have no floors, so when you sit down you have to brace your feet with great precision on either side of the hole. Beneath my boots I can see the gray snow rushing by, while music spews on the local radio.

At the student center, any request is submitted to the good will of the kommandante. So, on the day I decide I need to change rooms, I show up at her office with my heart pounding and sit down at the table facing her: "May I change rooms, please?" Her dour face stays impassive: "Nyet," she replies, pursing her lips. She's wearing a jacket that looks like a uniform, she has platinum blond hair and her cold, pale blue eyes cut through me without really seeing me. I repeat my question—"May I change rooms, please?"—but this time I bump her knee under the table with a box of Champs-Élysées chocolates. "Da," she replies, almost automatically, without smiling or so much as relaxing her mouth.

That very same evening, I'm in a new room, without any broken window panes.

I've never been happier.

Poets in Space

OCTOBER 2012. PARIS, KORIAN JARDINS D'ALÉSIA.

The red and gold leaves of the tall oak in front of the windows shiver. Fall has set the old tree ablaze.

When the television goes quiet in l'Espace, the dementia room, the cello starts to meander across the wilderness. In the summer, its music goes quiet in the warm, still air, and come fall it sings the wind in the trees, the snapping branches in the underbrush, the rain, the red leaves twirling down. We go strolling together, the cello and I. The round table in front of us is covered in dried leaves—gold, crimson, orange, and yellow, twigs, pieces of bark, and dirt, which we take turns touching, smelling; some people, for whom memory has erased the familiar sense of things, even taste or eat them. The cello mimics the ground cracking underfoot and the smell of roasted chestnuts, and words, sounds, gestures, and sensations long buried now emerge, bursting out everywhere to evoke autumn in poetry and in dance, like a canvas beneath the artist's agile paintbrush.

It smells delicious,
Leaves and mushrooms,
Dark bread,
Lovely chrysanthemums.
Snapping twigs,
Green moss,
Soft,
Unctuous,
Spongy,
Welcoming,
A deep love that slips away,
Memories.
Bring back that state of mind to me,
Full of hope,
The heart of the red autumn,
Light.

In spring, pale lips mutter about the "glorious, jubilant" season, and the wind is "warm, tremulous, turning yellow..." Summer, meanwhile, has a "warm heart, full of hope," fall is "grayish-purple melancholy," and winter looms with its "white moon, brown earth, black willow, the sun before us weeping, a dark happiness inside the heart."

Something simple and deep comes out of these fabulous poems by these writers-for-a-day. As fragile as a fledgling in springtime and more powerful than a victory cry.

We are happy
And we say it
We sing it
And we shout it.

The leaning woman stops walking, stands right in front of our table and watches us quietly. Her elbow pressed up against her waist, her head tilted, she comes to sit down with us for a few minutes.

The session—our celebration—has come to an end. The bells have been wrapped up, the drums and the maracas put away in the closet.

Madame Kessler, who has mixed dementia, is the philosopher. "Music speaks to something vital," she says, her voice quavering, "something essential within us, the most beautiful part of us. It transforms the person who is singing. It's a miracle."

Madame Olivier, who has schizophrenia, is more poetic: "We're not afraid of making mistakes here. We feel important now. We feel good. We feel at home."

Madame Renard, the painter, has Lewy body dementia. "Yes, we feel like we belong." She nods. "Alas, we must part."

Madame Beaurivage, the singer with Alzheimer's disease, was insulting her neighbors not an hour ago. "We sang well. We are coming away from this revived." "Yes," Madame Olivier adds, "what Madame Beaurivage says is true." Madame Beaurivage turns back to her: "You see, my dear, when you feel good, you're able to say it." And Madame Kessler answers, "You have a beautiful voice." Madame Beaurivage, in turn, replies, "Oh, but you are the one who recites so well." Monsieur Petit, who has Alzheimer's, never speaks. "You carry me under the surface of my ocean," he says now. "All the way down to the sand at the bottom. Down on the bottom." Madame Kessler concludes, "My dear, you're a wonder. Do you know why? Because you allow us to become wonderful again too."

Around the table, those who still understand words and those who have forgotten them nod their heads admiringly. They have truly become "travellers to unimaginable lands."

And although most of them will leave the room and immediately forget the cello, the bells and the drums, the strolls in the woods, the furtive caress of the wind, the swell of emotions and the kind words they've exchanged, it doesn't matter, because the attendants who are helping them back to their rooms are singing. An incomparable flash of light brightened the patients' faces for a few infinite minutes, and a glimpse of their flickering souls showed through, whole and intact. The stripping away, the dementia's successive theft is suddenly reversed, like some divine confirmation that, though some may say they are losing their minds, they have certainly not lost their spirit.

The heart is warm
And full of hope
Soon we will be happy
It's true
Together we dream
And our eyes light up

L'Espace, where the first-floor dementia patients spend their long days in this long room not of their choosing, has been transformed. What was empty space is now filled, and the bedridden patients now tread lightly on fine, golden sand on the linoleum floor.

The television won't be turned back on today.

The Moscow Conservatory

June 1993. Moscow.

For four years now, I've been working with the best teachers in Russia.

The Moscow Conservatory is a mythical place, haunted by the ghosts of composers like Glinka, Balakirev, Rimsky-Korsakov, and Shostakovich. My quartet and chamber teachers—my idols— are members of the Borodin Quartet, and they also become my adoptive Moscow parents.

My teacher, Marina Tchaikovskaya, who herself studied with the great Rostropovich, is teaching me how to play the cello. She worships her teacher, who fled the Soviet Union in 1974, and secretly hopes for his return. All those years, in every lesson, I hear her high-pitched voice: In the seventh measure of Brahms's Sonata in E Minor, Rostropovich said, you do an octave shift from E to E using the third finger; Rostropovich said, in the coda to the slow movement, put more weight on the baby finger on the bow, and especially narrow your vibrato; Rostropovich said…

Rostropovich becomes my teacher too, my model, my god in Russia and in the whole universe.

I barely get out alive. I don't care about the cold, the rats, the lineups in the stores, I want to learn and to get ahead, as much as I can. Madame Tchaikovskaya is dictatorial with her students, she pushes the cult of professionalism to the limit, she destroys students by humiliating them, subtly or extravagantly, depending on her mood that day.

"You don't know how to play... You don't know how to play at all."

"You don't even know what it is to be professional..."

"You don't understand anything anyway."

She turns me inside out, shattering me, and still I learn. I make enormous progress. I yield to her tyranny, even though I was brought up with such kindness, and I tolerate her reign of terror because I've encountered, or at least I think I have, what I've been looking for since my first cello lesson: a master who understands the instrument.

That understanding, that knowledge, is alive and impassioned, and it communicates an almost carnal relationship with the instrument, the technical command immediately generating an expressive response. In my classes, there is no dichotomy between technique and artistry, and it creates a musical gesture consciously rooted in the instrument, like alchemy.

I venerate her, I idolize her, she sculpts me and dismantles me at will.

Only much later will I understand that it is impossible to teach if you do not love.

The first year, I cry constantly. Every day, and often during my lessons, my tears drip onto my cello, they slide into the f-holes, leaving winding white salty tracks on the varnish, the measure of my abysmal imperfection.

"Do you know," she tells me, pointing to the other students in the class, who are sitting around on overstuffed couches listening to me curiously, "how many times they worked that shift from G to A?"

I am weeping miserably. I can't stop.

"Eleven years," she cries, "eleven years, for hours every day. And you, you've never done it, and you think you can get it just like that?"

Her face is scarlet and she scares me.

From two lessons a week, we go up to three. I work and work. I spend every day and late into the night playing a single open string, trying to acquire a round, even sound, that perfected, supple gesture. I practice far beyond what is reasonable, trying to master letting go of my weight in the right arm, trying to control the force of my fingers hammering on the fingerboard, analyzing the relationship between the vibrato's amplitude, speed, and pressure, in an insane attempt to be at one with the cello, and to create an authentic artistic expression.

I judge and I weigh every movement, every breath, every sensation. I love it. I suffer extraordinarily. I lose my mind a little.

A devastating feeling that I am worth less than nothing takes root within me, like a stem is pushing sharply through my chest, and I almost feel like I might die for not having reached my ideal—perfection.

A Musical Ballet

Bizet, *Carmen*
"L'amour est un oiseau rebelle" ("Habanera")

DECEMBER 2012. PARIS, KORIAN JARDINS D'ALÉSIA.

The leaves of the tall oak in front of the windows have fallen, floating slowly to the ground. The tree's branches are bare in the wind. Quietly, winter has settled in.

The concert is planned for three o'clock. There are posters throughout the building, on every wall. Downstairs, in the main hall, a crowd gathers—family members, friends, attendants. Upstairs, the excitement is at a fever pitch. Today's nap has been cut short to allow the performers to get dressed and do their makeup. Each person will wear a flower in their hair and a long, colorful cape adorned with the image of a white swan.

Over the course of five years, we have one hundred and twenty-two rehearsals around the round table, and nine public concerts. The residents are responsible for creating these multidisciplinary presentations.

The first concert is entitled "Love From the Earth to the Sky," spanning the musical repertoire on love, from the heavenly purity of a white sky conjured up by Gounod's "Ave Maria" to Bizet's *Carmen*, with the throb of springtime, love like a rebellious bird, the earth stained purple with blood.

The restricted-access elevator door is usually closed, but today—open sesame!—the artists go down one by one. The attendants arrange the wheelchairs in a semicircle in the already packed room.

The unlikely performance starts with the cello, though Madame Beaurivage's powerful voice soon swallows the instrument's sound and, without quite being aware of it, she leads all the others, the stuttering, the hoarse voices, the whispering voices, and the silent voices too. Charles Gounod, "Ave Maria." Ours is a strange unison. The sky is white with light.

Now the colorful silk scarves are twirling, tracing graceful arcs in the air. Eight artists, usually bedridden, dance madly without ever leaving their wheelchairs. Immobile bodies take flight. There is such joy on these furrowed faces. They look like lost angels, with bits of their wings swirling above their heads.

The attendants are dancing with the residents, and no one is really sure anymore who has become whose guardian angel.

Madame Kessler is an actress: she recites Maurice Carême, Baudelaire, Verlaine, and Rimbaud in a voice so vibrant that she is both the goddess and the muse in her own realm of tremulous words; she seems to have been the actual inspiration for the poetry.

The audience is speechless.

Now and then, a stray word sneaks in, pushing through the poem being performed. Madame Olivier begins to giggle uncontrollably and the poem derails, turns to shouts, and the choir of angels goes off-key and fades to an unintelligible murmur.

We worked so hard, and yet nothing goes as planned. The performers forget their parts, the carefully ordered program stumbles, and words flit off gleefully in transparent spirals.

The singer's lyrical phrase breaks off suddenly. Something is bothering her. Her blouse isn't buttoned straight. The audience waits, impatient. Just then, Madame Gazeau, who has never attended a single rehearsal, reaches out a trembling hand and rings the bell in an ascending scale that seems suddenly virtuosic, and the diva takes heart: Madame Beaurivage forgets her lopsided buttons, grabs a maraca as a microphone and, at the top of her lungs, lets loose that superb voice. The concert is back on—a triumph.

Madame Tisserand has been repeating everyone else's words constantly, catching a random word here and there, and her voice functions as the bassline of our unlikely orchestra, a seamless *perpetuum mobile*.

The handsome Monsieur Lemaître, meanwhile, is swinging. Madame Barthélemy's hands are fluttering like a swan as the cello sings Saint-Saëns, her crippled fingers beautifully evoking the migrating bird's wings, like a tear of white across the blue sky. Madame Rousseva, who is tetraplegic and who always sits out the rehearsals, is in the middle of the semicircle today, dressed up, her hair done, lying back in her wheelchair. They put her there by mistake. She has been paralyzed for two years, but her left toe is keeping the beat perfectly with the Bizet: "*L'amour est enfant de bohème.*"

She has a red flower in her hair. She is the queen of our concert.

The Turn

May 2007. Paris, 11th arrondissement.

Howard and I are sitting on the sidewalk terrasse of the café next to the Canal Saint-Martin. We're chatting about that day's miracles. Howard is staring at me with those eyes of his, as big as mountain lakes, the same eyes that took my measure ten years earlier in his dressing room backstage at the Ranelagh.

I've signed up for a university diploma program in art therapy at the faculty of medicine in Tours, but I don't want to talk about that with Howard. Starting those classes means challenging his almost biblical edict against learning anything about autism: "Surtout, ne rien lire." Whatever you do, read nothing.

"Howard, I want to study," I tell him, my voice shaky.

Howard goes quiet for a few seconds, which seem to drag on forever. Then, without so much as a smile, he says, "You won't learn anything, but you'll meet people."

Which is not completely true. But it is visionary in some ways.

By studying art therapy at the faculty of medicine, I will acquire professional status, I'll discover new definitions for my work, I'll learn tools and methods, strategies, the names for what I'm doing. I will ponder possible models for the link that exists between humans and art, but especially I will meet people.

Howard is right. I feel like he's always right. I'm going to meet doctors, attendants, patients. I will encounter or find again an undercurrent of confidence, the joy that pulsed through the wall that day between my bedroom and my beloved mother's.

A Day Like Any Other

Albinoni, Adagio in G Minor

JANUARY 2013. PARIS, KORIAN JARDINS D'ALÉSIA.

The leaves of the tall oak in front of the windows are piled in orderly heaps around the garden. The wind scatters them merrily.

In the small, cramped nurses' room, I'm sitting back during the change-of-shift meeting. Two attendants are dozing in their chairs, their mouths hanging open. It's nap time.

I take careful notes, as I do every week during the change-of-shift report. Something dull and uneasy lodges in my belly.

L. yelled all night. He woke up the whole floor. He finally calmed down two hours ago.

P. has been pacing around nonstop. She wanders into other residents' rooms and rifles through their closets. She stole some of S.'s blouses, and the family complained.

V. hasn't eaten in four days.

M. refuses to wash and throws himself to the ground when the nurses come to bathe him.

D. isn't moving anymore, but every morning she wants to jump out the window.

L. was found naked in T.'s bed.

B. tried to smother her cat under a pillow.

L. hasn't been able to hear anything since she was given some medication to unplug her ears.

F. is terrified of the night nurse.

M. calls everyone Master.

B. is very sad, and her companion is sadder still.

L. is aggressive. He whacks residents who are walking too slowly with his cane.

My pencil is shaking.

T. bit the night attendant so hard she bled, twice.

P. wants to marry her own son at the Christmas party.

The main characters in this parade are mostly the first-floor residents, the twenty-one patients with dementia, the artists of the room known as l'Espace. The term *resident* has always seemed strange to me. The implications of the word *dementia* are even worse.

That same day, I jot down the change-of-shift notes in my little notebook: "G. is no longer able to articulate words, he can no longer say no. He only says '*oui, ouiiii, ouiii.*'"

She and Him

Dancehall tango

FEBRUARY 2013. PARIS, KORIAN JARDINS D'ALÉSIA.

Room 208, room 209.

He has Alzheimer's, she has a Parkinson's-like neuro-degenerative disease.

His cognitive faculties are severely limited, but he's in excellent physical shape. Her mind is clear as a bell, but her body is completely paralyzed. They live together here, in adjoining rooms on the second floor. They have been married for forty-eight years.

She whispers to me, asking for tangos, waltzes, paso dobles—memories of the dance halls of their youth. He dances in front of her, holding her hands. She laughs, and weeps with happiness. There is no difference between her tears and her laughter. She lets herself dance with him without moving an inch in her high-tech medical chair. "Again... Again," she breathes, barely a murmur, as soon as the cello goes quiet. She feels herself flying through the past anew, though she struggles to convey that to me, her words subtle. He is happy. "This is good for my problems," he says, and he laughs loudly, agile as he dances forward and sideways.

Her eyes are sharp blue, two dazzling sapphires in a face made of glass. Her gaze is so transparent it looks like a gemstone, full of blue warmth. Her soul is nimble and huge in a fragile, crystal body.

He likes to lie down on his side to better savor the music. He has a funny way of dancing lying down. "That's pretty, that's good, that feels good here," he says, caressing his heart. "You make us happy." He rubs his index finger and his thumb together for a long time, as if he's trying to name an indescribable flavor. He looks at his wife: "It's like another world, and we're having a taste."

She blinks her eyelids quickly in agreement, whispers her thanks with enormous effort. The gems of her eyes are beaming. Her tense fingers relax and rest along her body. Her hands are open. During one session, she's almost able to unfold her arm. The coordinating physician makes a detailed report to the woman's family doctor.

One night, he goes into the neighboring room to look for her, and he can't find her. From then on, he looks for her in the hallway, in every room on the floor, searching them one by one, day and night. He waits. She left without a sound, somewhere far away, taking with her that bright blue of her eyes. He still wants to dance with her, he wants to taste the cello, as he puts it. A few weeks later, his own health deteriorates. He complains that he can't hear, and soon he's gone totally deaf. "I've gone deaf," he tells everyone he meets, waving his long hands; "somebody screamed, right in my ears... Tell me, have you seen my wife?"

Faculty of Medicine

October 2010. Tours, François-Rabelais University.

During my art therapy program, I discover the theoretical side of a practice that so far has been entirely intuitive for me. I learn the mechanics of "artistic interventions" and protocols, I establish case-based baselines, I try to define specific observation items—facial expression, eyes, attention, concentration, imagination, bodily involvement, residual motor skills and memory recovery, cognitive capacity, relational involvement—and measure each one for frequency and intensity. I draw up observation sheets, careful to note only perceptible, measurable facts about the patients. I've never worked like this before. My artistic soul is screaming for respite, but I submit to the process. Little by little, I start to absorb the data. I devour it, and I assimilate it. Faced with a pile of theoretical case studies, I track down and pinpoint the broken links of imaginary patients using analytical tools and grids. I spend hours quantifying smiles and eyebrows, deriving figures to plot on graphs. There are beautiful shapes in the colorful, skillfully calculated curves that overlap and intersect, and I would love to show them to Howard, but he's back at the center with the kids.

We could laugh together, we could dance with the children, tracing these surreal choreographies.

You're right, Howard, I'm not learning anything fundamental that I didn't already know. But, you see, I'm so much better equipped now to carry out and present my work, I can provide well-founded answers to questions, I can put my encounters into words. I can impress those who doubt me. I could impress you too, though you never once doubted me. I have plenty of quantitative evidence of the results of my work all laid out on giant slides. I'm being invited to serious conferences. And I can see you smiling: you're proud of me, because you know that my work, my approach, and especially my joy are still the same.

The Poet on the Second Floor

Johann Strauss, *Emperor Waltz*

MARCH 2013. PARIS, KORIAN JARDINS D'ALÉSIA.

The leaves of the tall oak rustle before the windows. Dressed up in their Sunday best, the branches, like arms, embrace an invisible friend. I think about that every time the wind blows through the tree.

The second-floor hallway is long, and the walls are covered in lemon-yellow wallpaper with large flowers that fold gracelessly over each other.

Madame Vaillant inches forward shakily, clutching her walker. "Get all these people out of here!" She shouts epithets at all the attendants who cross her path, the ones who wash her every morning. She's a small, skinny woman, hunched over, with an angular face. According to her file, she has Lewy body dementia, the symptoms of which include cognitive impairment and visual hallucinations.

"It's no good, no good." She stops, peeking around left and right like a little bird. Suddenly, she screams. "Help!" No one really pays any attention to her. Madame Vaillant has been banned from the dining hall for a week for stabbing her fork into her neighbor's arm at supper.

That day, I find her sobbing in front of the nursing station. "I can't go on, I can't take it anymore, I can't!"

I like planting my endpin in unexpected places. Any attendants who happen to be around tend to stop and put their grueling routine on hold for a few minutes. With great effort, Madame Vaillant is settled into a chair in the nursing room.

The *Emperor Waltz*, Johann Strauss.

Madame Vaillant blinks in surprise. After a moment, her sobs subside. She even seems vaguely amused and starts to clap before the end of the piece.

Madame Vaillant has no husband, no children, no friends. There's an older brother she expects every Sunday but who never comes. Her only possession—her armor, her pride, her defense against the world—is her National Order of the Legion of Honor, which was awarded to her on May 21, 1975, by Valéry Giscard d'Estaing.

"No good, no good": every Monday, when I come into her room, she greets me from the edge of her bed. "I'm going to die," she informs me.

Strauss's *Emperor Waltz*. Bach's gigue from the Cello Suite no. 2. The "Marseillaise." The cello sings with its warm, round, plaintive voice.

I note the phrases she repeats. During our next session, I hand her the fledgling poem she created, printed on a white sheet of paper in an ornate font.

It's no good
No good
I can't go on.

Have mercy
On me
I can't go on.

Have mercy
I don't know how
I'm lost now.

She's speechless. She reads the poem carefully a second time and looks up at me, her lips trembling a little, with an expression I've never seen before. "It's actually not bad!"

The next week's poem is called "My Anger, My Treasure."

Still sitting on the edge of her bed, she doesn't notice the attendant peeking through the half-open door, concerned suddenly that there isn't any screaming.

Bit by bit, week by week, words come to Madame Vaillant, mysteriously, enabled by my presence and the *Emperor Waltz*, Bach's gigue, and the "Marseillaise." It's like water gushing from an unseen mountain spring, so many rivulets pouring down that they spill into the valley and splash us both, so fresh we burst out laughing.

My anger is mute
Because I'm not allowed to speak.
My anger is grounded
Too heavy to fly.
I can't take it to supper:
There, they abhor me.
And I can't share it
Because they exclude me.

My anger is dark blue
And sharp as a spade.
My anger smells like soup left uneaten.
My anger is hungry.
My anger is mute.

I wouldn't want to leave it outside
For fear it might be taken.

Maybe I could bury it
In a hole.
Not too deep
Not too soft
To dig it back up again
If I had to
If I had to…
Take it back
And sell it
If I had to
If I had to.

The *Emperor Waltz*, Bach's gigue, the "Marseillaise."
Between pieces of music, she dictates and I write. I read it back
to her, again and again. She's concentrating. She surprises
herself. She is revealing herself. My presence makes hers
authentic and her words come alive as they shudder on the
edge of the pile of white paper.

The promise of future expression pulses within her like the
possibility of freedom.

A *Life*: The Book

APRIL 2013. PARIS, KORIAN JARDINS D'ALÉSIA.

This morning two branches are being chainsawed off the tall oak in front of the windows. The noise is deafening. It was dangerous for the residents, the receptionist tells me. Felled branches sit across the yard like huge emperors.

That day, Madame Vaillant and I decide together that we're going to write her autobiography.

The first interviews are painful. Madame Vaillant can't remember anything. Try as she might, nothing is coming back to her.

The *Emperor Waltz*. Bach's gigue. The "Marseillaise."

She listens without saying anything. She stares. Then there's a quick twinge, always the same, as if her pupils were twitching. Her eyes become animated. She doesn't interrupt my playing, but at the end of the piece, she says, "Wait." Her voice is nasal. "There's something coming back to me after all." A few scattered fragments emerge from her slumbering mind. The cello's voice calls up her memories, one by one. They hiccup forth and rise to the surface like rainbow soap bubbles bursting.

We may think things have been swallowed up or erased, but sometimes music can retrieve memories from hidden corners. Light flickers deep within the cello's chords. The strange feeling of being outside of yourself fades. Madame Vaillant can't exactly retrace the trajectory of her life, but we manage to connect the few pieces she lets through, enough to build a narrative. She was born in a village in Auvergne deep in the Cantal region, her parents were schoolteachers, she went up to Paris, she studied at the Sciences Po, the Paris institute of political studies. Then she started working, eventually got a job fairly high up at the National Education Ministry, and traveled to French Polynesia when the Loi Debré was applied to the overseas territories. In 1978, when she was secretary to education minister Christian Beullac, Madame Vaillant traveled to Jakarta with him. Turbulence rattled the small plane, and, as the panicked passengers clutched their armrests, the minister leaned over to her. "Don't worry," he said, "you'll get a state funeral." She tells the story over and over again, and every time it seems strangely disturbing to her, a shadow darkening her gaze like a light wind pushing the clouds across the sky.

Over eight months, I write down what she says. The book is coming along, and now we're looking for illustrations. Madame Vaillant has no strength left in her hands and legs, but she has an opinion on everything: no period here, put a comma here. Make sure the photo of her birthplace is centered. The flower necklaces in Nouméa are too pale. Couldn't we find another picture? Every week I show her the manuscript and she corrects it meticulously. She organizes the layout. She chooses the cover photograph, a view of the Sciences Po building on Saint-Guillaume street.

Whole sessions are devoted to the binding, the size of the book, the number of chapters, the size of the type, the grain of the paper. She's worried about the title, *A Life*: "I hope they don't say we copied Maupassant or Simone Veil." Madame Vaillant is well read.

"Maybe we could sell it," she suggests one day, but then immediately hedges: "Five euros, no more." As the book nears completion, she's sitting so tall in her wheelchair that all the attendants take notice. She takes their compliments graciously, smiling vaguely like the queen on an official outing. The book launch is set for May 25, 2014. We have to prepare a speech, to make sure the microphone works, pick an outfit. She only has one evening dress, a Chanel, which she last wore when she accepted her Legion of Honor forty years earlier. She refuses to have it cleaned because she's afraid, as she says, that "the maids will wreck it."

After ten months of preparation, the book is finally out in the world, but Madame Vaillant is so emotional that she is unable to utter a single word of her speech. The audience isn't paying any attention at all. The food carts clatter by back and forth at the back of the room. All the copies of *A Life* disappear in a few minutes in the pandemonium.

Madame Vaillant looks years younger. She's beaming with pride. That night, her exile is lifted, and she is allowed to return to the dining hall. Now that her neighbors know who she is, she says, she promises not to stab them with a fork. It doesn't matter if the book is only five chapters long, or that it contains no secrets or revelations. It doesn't matter if some people don't even know what the Legion of Honor is. She is both the author and the protagonist of her own story. She has become a different person, one whose story is worth telling, and who has taken the initiative, through the chaos of dementia, to spin a fabulous tale.

She's found new momentum within herself. She has recreated a sequence, a thread; she has reintroduced permanence. She has reclaimed the course of her life.

A Life, the book, prominently placed on the bedside table, is the only object in her room. She watches it greedily, moves it around. Sometimes she hides it because she's afraid it might be stolen. She takes it with her in a small bag tied to her walker when she shuffles to the dining hall twice a day. Her book is a trusted friend: it leads her gently by the hand along the yellow halls, it helps her into the elevator and to the table, and, at night, in her starless solitude, it stays by her side and comforts her.

Writing

1979, Paris, 16th arrondissement, Avenue du Président-Wilson.

"Yes, hello. Is this Éditions Gallimard?"

I've just called the famous publishing house number on my old rotary phone, the dial squeaking faintly. They transfer me politely from one department to another. After several minutes, which seem like forever to me, I hear a voice ask, "How old are you, Mademoiselle? I see... Very well... Send us your book. Make sure you include a summary as well. We're interested." Overjoyed, I skip around the apartment, I can't stop.

I'm twelve years old and I've just finished my first novel. I've been writing day and night on an old typewriter that belonged to my maternal grandmother, an American poet. The machine kicks out letters on the delicate legs of its strikers. The black ink ribbon is old, and some capitals—always the same ones—tear through the paper in a fitful, clanging dance. I write as soon as I wake up, the moment I get home from school, every spare instant I have. I fill my whole life with writing, so much it makes me *dizzy. I feel good when I'm surrounded by words; it's like there's a happy volcano of writing inside me. My novel is called* Clarisse. *It's a story of a young blind girl who gets her sight back. I love light even more than I love the night.*

Back then, I also loved the silence of words more than I loved the round, warm, plaintive sound of the cello.

Yet it is the cello's voice that will bring me back to writing so many years later. The movement of writing that is etched into the flesh, that transforms the mind and brings it beyond itself, with what silence and night it holds, folded into the light of encountering.

I never did finish that summary for Gallimard. And I never did send them my book.

The Legion of Honor Exhibit

Bach, Cello Suite no. 2 in D Minor, gigue

JULY 2014. PARIS, KORIAN JARDINS D'ALÉSIA.

The leaves of the tall oak in front of the windows are clad in their summer gowns, woven of silk and heat and storm.

Madame Vaillant and I still keep meeting after the launch of her autobiography. My repertoire is always the same: the *Emperor Waltz*, Bach's gigue, the "Marseillaise." Nothing else. It's ritualistic, and it holds the memory of that first appeasement, that first victory.

She's never held a paintbrush in her life, but at the beginning of the summer, she goes from writer to painter. Every Monday, an easel, brushes, a palette, and tubes of oil paints invade her night table. Together, the two of us patiently draw an insignia on the canvas, tracing it first in pencil. We paint her Legion of Honor: we shape and color its arrowhead arms, the proud head, the wreath. A white, five-pointed star, green laurel leaves, the crimson fold of the ribbon, Marianne's golden face, the medal sparkling on a black background.

At the end of each session, Madame Vaillant cries. My departure tears her apart. Her face tenses and she sighs, sharp words on the tip of her tongue.

A year later, Madame Vaillant puts on the Chanel dress again. Her vernissage is well attended and the common room on the ground floor is crowded. The exhibit has only one painting. Madame Vaillant is radiant.

After the party, the Legion of Honor in its gold frame stays on the wall for some time, and now and again, visitors or families notice it. Eventually we hang it in her room, nailed on the wall across from her bed. "It's beautiful," she says.

Musical Transfer

September 2015. Saint-Germain-en-Laye, Claude-Debussy departmental conservatory.

Maxime is nine years old. He stands in front of me clutching his cello with both hands. He is taking the entrance exam for the conservatory where I teach and has just played two short pieces for me. There are a lot of candidates this year, and already I know he won't get in. He's been playing for a year, and has too many technical flaws; I like starting students younger so I can train them from the start. I ask him a few questions about his background and thank him. As he's about to leave the room, I don't know what makes me ask him one last question: "What is it you want to do, with the cello?" He smiles. His face is glowing.

"Me? I want to play like Rostropovich."

In one second flat, Maxime becomes my student.

Maxime is a plant that never stops blooming. He is full of dreams and promise. His talent is so vast that he will accomplish in four years what few are able to do in twelve. He's never arrogant.

He works incredibly hard, with seemingly unwavering pleasure. He has no sense of time in his lessons: three hours go by as if it were barely ten minutes to him. He doesn't feel fatigue, even though he gets tired sometimes. His progress is spectacular and makes me think of bright, colorful, joyful petals opening again and again, week after week. His playing goes beyond technique, performance, or circus tricks.

In less than five weeks, he has adjusted his posture and his position. After three months, he's able to play simple pieces in public, with a round, warm, plaintive sound, which holds the promise of great maturity and deep musicality. In the four years that follow, he becomes a cellist. He wins every national and international competition he enters. His model, his only god, is Rostropovich. And I know what to tell him, I know what the master would have wanted, at least for some pieces, after gorging myself on Rostropovich too during my years in Moscow. The difference is that everything that was so painful during my training in Russia—the violence in so many interactions there, the fear, the humiliation—now has no place in this teacher–student relationship. What story do you want to tell, what do you want to express? How can you get there? What is your path?

I teach him to befriend his instrument, to be at one with the cello, to feel every vibration. I teach him to breathe, to project his sound by expanding the space around him, and to make every gesture open up a musical flourishing. I teach him to like scales *and the twinkle and taste of arpeggios just as much as the great works of the classical repertoire. He's delighted by every new étude; every sonata is an undiscovered land we cross together. He dreams of new concertos like faraway islands where we invariably wash ashore sooner than we thought. In the work of constructing the music, of binding form and content, in the journey and the destination, what brings us together is joy. Although it's hard, the relentless work is wholly devoid of suffering, and there is such an infinite, constantly renewed desire to learn, always looking toward beauty that shines out onto others.*

Through him, Moscow lives again, luminous.

Painting the Seasons

Handel, "Lascia ch'io pianga"

APRIL 2015. PARIS, KORIAN JARDINS D'ALÉSIA.

Heedless of the din on the street, the leaves of the tall oak in front of the windows never tire of the cycle of birth, life, death, and rebirth.

"I need a push," Monsieur Berger tells me when we start painting. "Maybe it's you?" This charming man, who used to be an ophthalmological surgeon, has vascular dementia. His wide bedroom window opens directly onto the oak in front of the residence. Together, we get to know the tree like it's a friend watching us from the yard, and we travel with it across the seasons. It's winter when we first paint the oak, its branches black and torturous. Spring cloaks it in tender green, and Monsieur Berger is filled with gratitude: "Tell my wife to go buy me lots of greens," he cries when he sees me come in, "light green for now, and dark green in a few weeks."

As I'm getting ready to leave, he says, "I don't dare ask, but I would love you to come more often... You are my resurrection! You're a kick in the pants! You're a ray of light!"

After a sweltering summer, we dip our brushes into the red and the gold and spend whole weeks spreading the burnishing leaves over the rasp of the canvas as they fly off the tree, watching in silence as the wind ruffles the big oak's foliage. "I'd like to paint the wind," he tells me one day. "I'd like to make the invisible visible in my paintings. Shall we try?"

Handel's "Lascia ch'io pianga": let me weep. The music courses through him like fire. "There's a deep echo inside me. You have to know how to listen." He closes his eyes. "It's like a current. I'm not trying to be a philosopher, it's not literature, you know, I'm just trying to feel the vibrations that touch me. Every time, I learn something, in my flesh. My sense of taste vibrates. The deepest places within me move and recalibrate, like a silent echo."

Meanwhile, in my head, I quietly thank this old man, my wise friend, who better than anyone is able to express what I feel, what I've always felt, which led me to him, to all of these people. And to myself.

A sense of trust.

The purveyance of joy.

In the Metro

May 2001. Paris, a metro car on line 5.

"You don't think they look strange?"

It takes me a moment to understand that Howard is talking about the other passengers who are in the metro with us. We've just left the Adam Shelton Center. Djamel scratched Howard's forehead, his cheek, and his right eyelid. He looks like he's just had his makeup done for a new show. I watch the tired after-work crowd.

Howard is pensive.

"If something happens to me one day," he says, as if this followed logically from his preceding observation, "I would want you to come play for me."

Howard says unexpected, inscrutable things.

Leading Lady

Schubert, Piano Trio no. 2 in E-flat Major, op. 100
Development

MAY 2015. PARIS, KORIAN JARDINS D'ALÉSIA.

Madame Kessler is getting weaker. She's been in her wheelchair all the time. All day long and all night, she moans. Her voice no longer carries when she speaks, and her diction is altered. Months go by, and she can't read the poems anymore, even though I increase the font size. One day, she speaks only German; no one knows why.

And yet each time the cello sings, tremors of joy still run through her body, from top to bottom. That spring afternoon, I find her among our companions at the table, sobbing and unable to say a single word.

I begin to tell them a story, the story of the Schubert treatment. *Once upon a time*, the story begins, *there was a great* woman, *Madame Kessler, a magnificent artist who was suffering tremendously. One day, miraculously, her pain was relieved by the andante from Schubert's Piano Trio, played for her on the cello.* I recount the scene in detail—that first treatment in the common room, then the clinical study at Sainte-Périne hospital. The media caught wind of this new nonpharmaceutical approach and it started making the rounds at medical conferences in France, Spain, Switzerland, Canada, Japan, Israel. Madame Kessler is immobile in her wheelchair, and although she is racked by pain and anguish, she beams with pride at hearing the story. The others around the table are listening. Some don't quite get it, but most of them start clapping, as pleased as she is at the idea that she's become the heroine of a story, which after all is their story too.

A New Place

January 2011. Paris, Sainte-Périne hospital palliative care unit.

Dr. Jean-Marie Gomas is a creative physician, a crusader. The first time we meet, he trusts me immediately. He is extremely open to my project of providing live music for therapeutic purposes in his unit.

Since 1995, he's been at the helm of a first-rate palliative care program, which he created and has developed over the years in a public hospital that specializes in geriatrics. As he points out, the service is available for adults from eighteen to one hundred and twenty years of age.

He never doubts me for a second. He believes in bringing the power of music within his care team, and for years he's been hoping to meet an artist and therapist who could bring to life his vision for working with patients in end-of-life care.

My approach views patients holistically, trying to reach a critical aspect of what it means to be human—our sensitivity to art, our creative capacity, our imagination. Jean-Marie is full of *projects and ideas. The next day, he's already reorganizing the schedule to allow me to work with patients on the ward. He fights like a lion to defend the new program to everybody—patients, families, the team, colleagues, the hospital directors. He's loyal and generous, and he's never afraid to say what he thinks. He knows how to convince others, and he knows how to listen.*

At the end of my six-month internship as part of the art therapy program at Tours, Jean-Marie suggests that the association he founded put me on salary so I can come in once a week and keep working with the patients.

Before long, I find myself immersed in the world of conferences and scientific publications.

Howard forbade me from reading, while Jean-Marie pushes me to research.

Howard privileges intuition, while Jean-Marie encourages analysis.

A year and a half after I start working in the palliative care unit, I present the results of my music therapy sessions to a medical conference in Paris. It's the first time my cello and I are speaking to a room full of doctors and caregivers. The emotion in the room is palpable.

This is a turning point for me.

"You'll have to come back for the Schubert treatment," the nurse said to me in the common room after Madame Kessler was miraculously appeased that first day.

I ended up going back one hundred and twelve times.

At the Sainte-Périne hospital palliative care unit, the andante from Schubert's Piano Trio helps mitigate one hundred and twelve painful treatments: baths, dressing wounds, oral care, agonizing mobilizations, blood tests, and abdominal taps.

The Schubert treatment makes me a caregiver.

I feel like I've found my place.

Monsieur Roy's
Blood Test

Bach, Orchestral Suite no. 3 in D Major, aria

MARCH 2013. PARIS, SAINTE-PÉRINE HOSPITAL.

Room 410 in the palliative care unit, spacious and bright, opens onto the garden.

On March 29, at exactly three o'clock in the afternoon, I set up in a corner of the room by the door. Monsieur Roy arrived yesterday. Seventy-four, metastatic colon cancer. He's suffering from severe anemia, and he's having cognitive issues. He often aspirates and stops breathing. He was a hard poke, the nurses said yesterday: extremely difficult venous access due to the patient's movements. He was frightened, crying and fighting. His arms are bruised black and blue from previous venipuncture, and yesterday it just wasn't going to happen.

Monsieur Roy is lying on his bed, and, in spite of his obvious anxiety, he's looking at me out of the corner of his eye, looking slightly surprised. It was fine, he said. Yes, he likes music. What's that? The cello is from the eighteenth century? He's never seen such an old instrument. The nurses are prepping.

I begin with Schubert, the andante from the Trio no. 2. The cello's warm, round, plaintive voice vibrates around the room. One of the attendants starts humming. She adjusts the needle and gently touches the patient's arm. He tenses. But Schubert sings and the melody dives low for a few measures, rolling like waves on the sea. The nurse brings the needle closer, and as she slides it in, precise and efficient, Schubert swells, climbing back up the scale. Instead of screaming like he did the day before, the patient begins to sing too; he is even conducting with his right hand. The nurses look at each other and burst out laughing. The blood fills the vial quickly. Monsieur Roy is inspired now, a conductor leading my cello and his orchestra with sweeping arms. His face is relaxed and his eyes twinkle.

He begins to sing so loudly that an attendant passing by pushes the door open, worried. They're done with the blood test, but he keeps conducting. "Okay, Monsieur Roy, all done." His imaginary baton stops in midair. "Well, look at that." He realizes what's just happened. "That was easy as pie today." The nurses are smiling and swaying slightly as they put their things away. Monsieur Roy is beyond pleased, and he says so with gravitas and finesse: "That was enchanting. More than just the heart, music touches the soul, and all the pain flies away."

This is the first experiment in the Schubert treatment clinical trial: sensory counter-stimulation during a painful procedure in palliative care.

Clinical Trials

Starting in April 2013, the clinical study is implemented by the whole care team. The primary therapeutic objective is to reduce pain and anxiety during unpleasant nursing procedures, notably blood work. The study has quite naturally been dubbed the Schubert treatment. The initial project includes the study of two hundred Schubert treatments over three years.

Treatments with and without cello accompaniment will be compared on alternating days in order to observe the extent to which live music's sensory counter-stimulation has a beneficial impact on the procedure as a whole and on patient pain and anxiety, but also on the psychological health of caregivers and family members.

My university studies are incredibly useful here. For the first time, I connect my intuitive approach and a theoretical process. I dive deep into the research. I have the tools to try to assess possible improvements in patient symptoms, even though the source of those improvements remains by nature immeasurable and indefinable.

Every contextual and methodological element is explicitly laid out: patient population, pathologies, cognitive issues, possible changes in vision and hearing, adapted verbal capacities, psychotropic and sedative impact on communication, degree of responsiveness and communication, type of procedure, pre-medication, number of caregivers per session, duration, patient proclivity for art, adapted musical repertoire.

With the support of the Centre national de ressources de lutte contre la douleur, the national pain management resource center, we implement a Schubert treatment observation chart, detailing specific clinical parameters to note and compare prior to, during, and following each procedure. These charts are a record of the events, and allow for data collection. The exercise is quantified, analytical, and exact, an accurate way to assess the activity.

Jean-Marie contacts various foundations, looking for funding to carry out the study. Families whose loved ones have benefited from the sessions make donations to an association set up for the purpose. As for me, I'm completely involved with the caregivers, working with the multidisciplinary team, available every week for every patient on the unit.

Madame Moretti's Bath

Gluck, *Orpheus and Eurydice*, melody

MAY 17, 2013. PARIS, SAINTE-PÉRINE HOSPITAL.

Madame Moretti, seventy-eight years old, has metastatic cancer. She was admitted to palliative care yesterday, uncomfortable, in pain, and nonresponsive.

I'm sitting at the nursing station with the care team for the change-of-shift meeting. The nurses are telling us how hard it was to turn the patient in her bed yesterday when they bathed her because her limbs are so stiff and tense. The doctor immediately ups the morphine, along with increased injectable sedation prior to the procedure. The patient will have relief before our meeting is even over.

This team meeting happens every day, in the middle of the day. I take part on Thursdays. It's a crucial meeting: everyone listens, shares information, and discusses strategies and adaptations. I learned quickly that the palliative care unit is among the rare departments in the hospital where the medical team sits down every day with the care team. Jean-Marie insists on that sacred time, like a ritual, as a way to make sure a seasoned team is providing personalized care to each patient.

When I sit down in room 404, between the white-uniformed nurses crowding together I see Madame Moretti's emaciated face, tense with pain and the apprehension of pain. The attendants set out tubs of warm water for her bath, and I begin to play. First Schubert sings as an overture, as an homage to Madame Kessler, then the melody from Gluck's opera *Orpheus and Eurydice*. Fragile resonance; an invisible caress. Again, that day, the presence of the cello affects the treatment. Madame Moretti's stiff, splayed fingers relax slowly and unfold one by one, and soon her hands are resting alongside her body. Beneath the white sheet, her feet drop apart from each other like the petals of a water lily opening to the sun.

Her face softens. The ridge on her forehead smooths out like sand after the ebb of a wave. Several times, Madame Moretti opens her eyes, revealing a bright, quick gaze. For a few moments, there is no pain. She can't say it in words, but her entire body announces it. Her muscles are so relaxed it's spectacular.

The nurses tell the two doctors who are there that morning about the cello session: "The patient smiled several times throughout the procedure. And she opened her eyes four times. It was obvious she appreciated the music. Her whole body relaxed, and her arms especially were incredibly relaxed. Totally different from yesterday's bath."

They describe their own emotions in the chart, too: "We were more focused on the procedure, and happier too. We felt harmonious together."

This is the second procedure in the clinical trial for the Schubert treatment.

Research

Our work is moving along. During the fall of 2013, we flesh out our observations using precise, targeted clinical parameters before, during, and after the treatment. The chart includes different pain scales, respiratory frequency, chest expansion, facial expression, body movements, position changes during treatment, and muscle relaxation, as well as an overall description of the procedure and of the emotional states of the patient and caregivers. Nurses fill out the information at the end of each session with and without music. It does create additional work; every Schubert treatment requires nursing staff to anticipate and reorganize their care protocols to some extent.

Some of the staff are less enthusiastic about this new approach, and one person in particular is downright opposed, which undermines the team dynamic for a while. There are also some who, although they're open to the approach, unconsciously feel that it implies a failure on their part, as if their care alone were not enough. There are cases in which improvements aren't obvious and the patient doesn't seem to react to the music, so that any relief provided is purely for the caregivers.

Over time, the care team evolves, and so do I. The organization of nursing care and the cello sessions becomes more sophisticated. This nonmedical approach is the subject of an open, comparative, nonrandomized prospective study, and the analgesic efficacy of the Schubert treatment is scientifically confirmed, rigorously so, albeit with the full awareness of limitations and possible biases. Our results are presented at international medical conferences in France, Switzerland, Spain, Canada, Japan, and Israel.

Mostly, and most importantly, on days when the cello sings along to painful procedures, there is a lot of joy on the unit. "We yell at each other less on Thursdays," the care team says.

The nurses are unanimous: the pain caused by the various nursing procedures and interventions is reduced by the music. They feel like they are being accompanied by something that doesn't quite belong to their field of work, yet which renews their perspective thoroughly, taking their emotions into account as well. They report a greater sensitivity to their patients' humanity, to the afflicted, and they say they feel more serene and gentle in their work. Their ability to express their emotions has improved considerably, and they also report finding "more courage to dare to be ourselves."

The Schubert Treatment

At first glance, live music seems like an intruder in the patients' rooms. Yet it does not damage or destroy; it is never shocking. It slips in and takes its place simply, always different and always the same, in this world of care, with pans of soapy water, gloves, syringes, forceps, and compresses. It doesn't matter whether it's Albinoni's Adagio or Joe Dassin's "Indian Summer," "My Yiddishe Momme," or a traditional Arab tune—for a few moments the music opens eyes that have been closed for a long time, it relaxes hands twisted and clenched in pain. Sometimes it lights up the patients' eyes and puts a smile on their faces or makes them cry, even when they're no longer conscious. Hearing live music makes patients on the threshold of death sing and dance, and the caregivers too come into the dance.

It opens every heart.

Bitter Medicine and the Breath of Music

FOR YEARS, SCHUBERT ACCOMPANIES various nursing procedures. Some are fluid and light, others difficult or complex, but
in almost every single case the music soothes and relieves the
patients, their families, and their caregivers.

During paracentesis, a procedure to drain excess fluid from
the abdomen, Monsieur D., in room 409, is singing "My Way"
with the nurses.

That morning, his bloated belly, which seemed about to
explode, relaxes as it empties painlessly. My 1749 Italian cello,
smiling with every fiber of its being, mingles with their voices.

"There are days when it's worth it. There's something to
hold on to," he says at the end of the session.

All music can be good and even beautiful.

Madame S., in 407, needs a dressing. She has soft-tissue sarcoma, which has left a deep wound on her thigh, the flesh so grisly that even the nurses falter for a second as the compresses are sucked into the lesion. For the first time since my arrival on the ward, as I am playing the French pop song "L'Aziza," a wave of nausea washes over me.

Only then do I understand the extent of my connection with the other caregivers, and my fragility, my limits.

There's a bed bath and shampoo in room 410 for Madame D., an ALS patient who, although pleased with the prelude to Wagner's *Die Walküre*, expresses her discomfort from time to time during the treatment—"This is hardly discreet!" Later, after rolling out her own vocalizations like a Wagnerian diva, she turns to me. "It is pretty funny, though, the intimacy of these ablutions, with high opera... *Oh là là!*"

And so I discover how close modesty is to laughter.

A bed shower in room 402 for a young cancer patient, Madame H., who has just arrived from Togo. She sings Schubert's "Ave Maria" on a loop with my cello, her hands clasped and her face beaming, as if she were gazing into her own soul. "It elevates me. It's just what I need: a piece of heaven."

I experience music as prayer.

Monsieur F., in room 406, needs a dressing for a sacral ulcer. He's a sedated, noncommunicative patient who listens to Albinoni's Adagio with fat tears running down the gray marble of his face.

The nurses and I are emotional too, unsteady, as if waves were battering our hearts.

A dressing for Monsieur T. in room 405, a patient in the final moments of his life. His wife sits behind me, whispering what music he loved in my ear. She is no longer allowed to wash her husband, but through the music she chooses, she's able to reconnect with the things she used to do for him at home.

Sound transforms before my eyes into a tender caress, one last kind touch.

Monsieur V., room 409, has complex needs. He's a chronic pain patient who is usually reluctant about or even dead set against any kind of care. Now he stops being aggressive. To the gentle adagietto of Mahler's Symphony no. 5, he lets the nurses take him in their arms like a child and return him to his bed. The nurses note, "Monsieur V. allowed himself to be carried away today with the cello. He even stroked our hands without pushing us away. His eyes were clearly saying 'thank you.'"

Silently I share the unsettling experience of watching a person trust another again, as if they were a newborn.

A bath for Madame R., a nearly mute cancer patient in room
404 who spills her monstrous story in a single breath after a
change of dressing to Handel's *Rinaldo*, revealing unspeakable
things. A wound deeply buried gives way to a rush of words
after the rush of sound.

I discover music beyond words as a possible way to set
words free.

Monsieur H.'s festive treatment, in room 401, when the
nurse and attendant start dancing with him to the beat of a
Cuban salsa. He can't get out of his bed, but can he ever move!
"Thankfully we still have music to save us! And your hair is
beautiful, too!" The care team notes, "The cello today was like
laughing gas. We were all laughing, including the patient. A
relaxed atmosphere. Monsieur H. danced with his feet. The
bath went very well."

I throw myself in wholeheartedly to celebrate the sudden
explosion of shared, rhythmic, bodily joy.

Monsieur N., a verbose patient in a lot of pain, needs a
patient-controlled analgesia pump installed, room 405. "It
hurts so much, it hurts. I can't take it, I can't take it anymore."
The cello's singing moves the patient, and his son and grand-
son, who are there too, and binds them together. All three of
them cry, pressed against each other, like a sculpture, racked
by suffering. I know their grief is bottomless and music can't

do much for them, yet it's strangely comforting. Everyone in the room feels it. I also know that it's not me personally who makes these moments so tender.

I'm so grateful to be able to give the gift of relief.

Monsieur C.'s bed bath and shampoo, in room 408. He's a cancer patient with bone and pulmonary metastasis. He is in a coma. The care team notes, "Massive increase in expansion of the chest cage while music was playing. Excellent experience for nurse/attendance team, a feeling of sharing or even communion between us."

The silence is filled with music that is louder than the music itself.

Monsieur F., in room 402, is at the very end of his life. His face, already incredibly relaxed, eases even more at the end of the session, into what the care team calls a rapturous expression. His son comes in at the end of the bath. "My father will be so full of life when he goes," he says. The nurse notes, "The patient is drowsy with eyes closed and slow response, but obviously relaxed. It took my own stress away. I was moved too. The music touched the emotional core of everyone in that room."

I learn that death and love roll in the same deep waters.

A change of dressing for Monsieur C.'s necrotic leg, room 407. He loves listening to top-forty hits from the sixties.

When the nurse asks whether she's hurting him, he shouts, "Shut up, I'm listening!" At the end of the treatment, he confides to the nurses with a smile, "How sweet that was. It felt good. I feel like I traveled far."

And I take part, as I do every time, in the invitation to travel.

Madame J., in room 409, needs a bath, and some fairly complicated repositioning. As she listens to the cello, she starts to cry: "It's beautiful. It's magical. She's good, the little pianist." Later, she asks, "Can you turn down the radio, please, sir?"

At the end of the treatment, as the nurses are spraying lavender on her sheets before leaving, she complains: "Can't you turn it off now? I've had quite enough."

I leave too—a piano virtuoso, a switched-off radio.

Monsieur H. needs a dressing. He looks worried when he sees me and pats his pajama pants, looking for money: "I don't have any change on me, or a bank card, sorry." When he is told that my playing won't cost him a penny, he's reassured, and changes his tune. "It's up to you, I have all the time in the world. Let's play some music!" A little while later, he seems downright charmed: "Say, darling, weren't we at the concert together? You're not from Turkey, are you, with that blond hair of yours?"

Inside I'm laughing so hard I'm crying. "Thank you," I tell him.

There are some treatments for sedated or comatose patients where the benefits of music are impossible to judge.

Some patients refuse to try or choose not to repeat the experience of being treated with music.

Some people, even the caregivers sometimes, are annoyed, sad, or even angry when the cello isn't there and they are, as they put it, abandoned.

Results

The results of one hundred and twelve Schubert treatments, published in 2016, demonstrate a reduction in patient pain ranging from ten to fifty percent. Positive effects on patient anxiety are assessed at approximately ninety percent. The positive effect on caregivers is one hundred percent.

The research does reveal to us the limitations of scientific study. Our study is first and foremost based on shared emotions that defy quantification, and as we work to reduce symptoms of pain in patients, our respective and often divergent subjectivities unquestionably also affect the analysis of that impact.

At a 2017 international palliative care conference in Geneva, I present an analysis of our methodological challenges. It's no simple thing to conduct evaluations using pain scales over extremely short periods of time, and to separate the effect of music from that of increases in analgesics or sedatives. I also mention the emotional bias music creates, which interferes with qualitative evaluation.

The whole adventure raises so many questions. What is the link between the vibrations of the instrument and the deep vibrations of the human patients; what kind of resonance is that? Does music create emotions, or does it reveal them? Is it possible to measure the level of apprehension of patients in palliative care? Can emotion be measured and feelings structured in an arithmetic grid without the whole exercise becoming absurd?

The bias of the assessors, who also make up the care team, is significant. The caregivers are at once observers and participants, carrying out a project that inherently includes a considerable positive suggestive effect. Yet that effect, instead of representing a confounding factor in the evaluation or even a major methodological bias, seems like a dynamic force, a veritable driver of care.

The Schubert treatment enables an unlikely meeting between medicine and live music, tinged with grace, during painful nursing procedures. It highlights a renewed relationship between the patient, their family, the caregiver, and the music therapist.

The music that resounds in the room speaks to what is alive and healthy in the patient, even if that part of them is only an infinitesimal speck of life and health.

Throughout my journey as a concert musician redirected toward medical care, I am sometimes a researcher, digging deep—I identify the phenomenon, pointing to it—and sometimes I'm just a companion, walking, and feeling, alongside.

The researcher tends to quantify, classify, analyze, prove. She points out the unmistakable objectivity of symptoms. She seeks to impose order on the observations.

But the companion neither directs nor controls. She doesn't need to know everything or apply any rules. The companion supports the irreducible individuality of the other. She is all presence and solidarity.

The poet must leave a trace, not evidence, wrote René Char.

The results of the Schubert treatment walk that fine line between scientific evidence and an artistic trace, a lasting memory of an invigorating, unifying experience for those who are ailing.

Monsieur Koumba

"I'm in the ring."

2011–2019. PARIS, SAINTE-PÉRINE HOSPITAL.

"When you play your cello, I get to rise up above my disease," Monsieur Koumba tells me one sunny spring morning. "I don't feel like I'm sick anymore." He trails off, waits a moment, grasping. "No," he goes on, "that's not it. When you play, I am actually not sick anymore. I feel happy, I feel alive." He speaks slowly, his breath halting, his neck stiff, drawn down into his shoulders. His eyes sparkle with laughter in his somber face. He requests another piece, and another.

Around the time I meet him, he is in a respite care program in the room set aside for ALS patients.

He noticed the disease a year earlier, when his legs became paralyzed. It progressed rapidly, to his torso, then his arms.

Monsieur Koumba is sixty-five years old. He is still able to move his hands—enormous, a champion's hands.

His breathing is labored, and at night he has to wear an oxygen mask to avoid suffocating in his sleep. He's a former boxer turned security guard. "I'm a bouncer," he says with a wink. He is still young. He is originally from Togo. A glorious, international athlete. His body now is leaden, completely inert.

Every time I see him, music transfigures him and inspires him to speak. He pronounces his words slowly, like an ancient sage, broken up by raspy inhalations: "Claire... Claire... This is an eternal experience... The body waking. Powerful... What you give me stays in me and it amplifies life." Memories abound as he listens to the cello. "You bring me back in time," he says. "Stay hopeful. Don't let go. Keep fighting... I can feel life... Life, until the very end..."

He nods solemnly.

Of all the patients I work with, he's probably the one who is able to articulate most accurately the singularity of these moments of music in a hospital room—moments that feed us, not just present, past, and future, but all of it mixed up together: "It's like I'm experiencing the deep past and the future at the same time." He is smiling, beaming. "I forget the present, I forget that I'm suffering. The past comes alive again, and the future opens up. It's a miracle, you know. The miracle of love and music. It gives me strength inside." He clasps his powerful hands, hands so soft, those heavyweight hands that swallow mine completely when we shake hello. "My friend, the great boxer Marcel Cerdan, he got everything, glory and love, but God took it all away." I never ask him questions. He loves all kinds of music, but he always wants to hear Édith Piaf, especially "Non, je ne regrette rien." He insists on taking off his oxygen mask during that song, and, out of breath, his face alight, he sings along, swinging his head right to left, never taking his eyes off me. "I'm in the ring," he concludes at the end of every song. "I'm strong enough to fight!"

Music is strength.
It weaves together sound and silence,
Gathers fragments of time,
And restores the permanence of being.
It summons the taste of the present,
Reaches the depths
And touches them, exalts them.
The ordeal of the life force
In a frozen body,
The return of intensity,
Of fluidity once more.

Madame Müller

"Sound-friends."

"MY CRY OF FEAR AT DEATH has been released into a sea of sound-friends! Oh dear… I couldn't help myself." Madame Müller bursts into tears at Albinoni's Adagio, which I play for her on the cello.

This forty-seven-year-old patient, who has breast cancer with hepatic and bone metastases, is hospitalized in the palliative care unit. Madame Müller always has a smile on her face. Always. She has soft brown eyes, and her skin is very pale. "I can't tell a lie, when it vibrates like that, it's so pretty. The music comes for me in secret places. It makes me cry out from the inside. Nobody else knows me like that." She mutters these words as if to herself, in sentences that are increasingly muddled through her tears. What I make out is her terror in the face of death; today, Albinoni's Adagio has released that cry in a "sea of sound-friends," rather than the indifferent silence of the everyday. I have a hard time understanding what she's saying. She clutches my hands, holds me back. "The Adagio, again, please…" She's abandoned her serene, smooth mask, and an expression of infinite anguish furrows her face, a strange contrast with the full roundness of her features.

So I play again and again. "Thank you for these sound-friends, they do me a world of good." Silently I thank her for having named the sounds of my beloved instrument like that. Just as I am leaving, she whispers without looking at me, "The sound-friends are welcoming me."

Music is a friend.
The sound-friends allow
A cry of terror in the face of death to burst forth.
They meet the scream,
Wrap it in mysterious echoes.
They enfold the cry in an invisible caress
that sometimes drowns it out.
The sound-friends try to hold at bay
That last letting-go foreseen and feared.
They comfort what cannot be comforted in its
unfathomable suffering
For an instant, brief and eternal.

Monsieur Rivière

"My hands can't clap, but my heart is cheering."

THE FIRST TIME I offer to play for him, Monsieur Rivière stammers an apology: he doesn't know what tune to choose. "I'm not an educated man," he says, worried, almost distraught. He has metastatic esophageal cancer, and was admitted three days earlier. He's a man in his seventies, with a gray complexion. He moves slowly. When I sit beside his bed and begin Bach's First Cello Suite he watches my fingers on the strings carefully. His eyes are soft and bitter, he's lost in unknowable thoughts. He seems to be daydreaming. I can almost make out the little flicker of sound-friends swirling around us in the room, twirling, spiraling invisibly through him.

His wife sobs next to him. I feel like the whole room is simultaneously ablaze and intensely calm. As I play the last chord, he looks up at me and says slowly: "This happiness is going to keep echoing. Your cello is vibrating, it's amazing. I'm touched." The clarity of his thoughts stands in contrast to his erratic diction. He's still hesitant: "I don't know much, but I can feel it."

Our sessions feel festive. Monsieur Rivière describes himself as full, supported; he's master of his domain again, he says. His wife cries. "My tears comfort me, they cleanse me," she says. "It does me good."

But each week Monsieur Rivière is getting weaker. His wife never leaves his side, not even at night: she sleeps next to him on a cot. The fourth time I see him, he has to make a huge effort to open his eyes and speak even a single word, but he insists on describing what he's feeling: "It fills me... Whole... Renews me. Gives life to my soul again. My hands can't clap, but my heart is cheering."

He is full of gratitude, and it still shows in his eyes.

The last sentence Monsieur Rivière speaks to his wife, on the eve of his death, is a gift, an offering, a whispered treasure that music sometimes bestows at death's door: "Living keeps on going, even when it stops."

We must name the splendor of things to try to live again.

Music is life.
The instrument's vibrations
Weave through to the heart's very core,
A place beyond words suddenly revived.
Life leaps,
A single movement in the broken body.
Music offers itself up entirely
To those who claim not to understand.
It speaks to the intelligence of the heart.

Monsieur Lebrun

"Could Rachmaninoff save me?"

MONSIEUR LEBRUN, a former intelligence agent, is hospitalized with metastatic prostate cancer. One side of his body is
paralyzed, and he can no longer get out of bed. Day and
night, despite powerful drugs, he complains that he feels a
pin sticking into his back. He has hallucinations that make
him extremely agitated, which is worsened by the fact that he
is almost completely blind, his eyes dulled by an opaque veil.
He is wan, his cheeks hollow. But this morning, when I play
Rachmaninoff's "Vocalise" for cello and piano for him, he says
to me, with great gentleness, "How strange it is that I'm the
same man who was lying in a cradle just a few years ago."

On the wall of his room a crooked black-and-white photo
shows a young man holding a small child in his arms. I can

make out some resemblance between the two slightly blurry figures locked in the photograph's eternal embrace.

When I stop playing, he feels for my hands and squeezes them. "As long as I can hear a cello playing, I will feel okay." After a long silence, he asks, "Do you also play for funerals?"

The following week, he hears that I'll be playing at the Russian embassy that evening. He holds out both hands to me again: "I want to come. Take me with you, please." He waves me closer to him, and whispers in my ear. "I have things to tell them..."

Our sessions are a form of shelter for him, a sanctuary in the ordeal, a safe space for memories to emerge, and a place of possible joy, too. He articulates all of this wonderfully. He is a poet. He touches me deeply. After each melody I play, he spins out something from his past, like a child plucking the petals of a wildflower, as the memories unfurl vividly, in full color, before his sightless eyes. He tells me about starting out in a British insurance company, and joining the army, then the police, then the French intelligence service. "Not bad, for a kid who was a bit of a loser," he adds with a smile.

Monsieur Lebrun is lulled by the music like a child cuddled up against their mother's heart. He wants the music to never stop, and he tries to prolong the resonance by whispering to me. "That ending, how the 'Vocalise' unravels like that. It slides right into me, it runs through me. It makes me feel good inside. Could Rachmaninoff save me?"

Rachmaninoff overwhelms him, moves him, makes him tremble, and, for a few seconds, lets him forget the pin he feels stabbing into his back.

"If you came every day, I could live more."

Music is vibration.
The instrument is a singer, it shudders, enfolds,
Seeps into the screaming body.
The ordeal of the life force,
The shivering past emerges
As a delicate trickle or a torrent, impetuous,
Dragging along all the buried emotion.
In that pulse, during the breath of a vocalise,
The feeling of existence
Takes on the flavor, full and sweet,
Of childhood.

Monsieur Martin

"It's still good."

MY FIRST ENCOUNTER with Monsieur Martin is sharp, almost aggressive. He's seventy-five and has lung cancer with bone metastasis. He is a short, stocky man who used to own a café in the suburbs of Paris. When I suggest I play some music, he throws me a nasty look. "Damn thing," he pants. "It hurts. Why am I so tired? I don't care about music." But as I turn to leave, he retracts: "Why don't you give it a try. We'll see." I sit down in front of him and play the first notes of the Léo Ferré song "Le Temps du tango." His face stiffens.

C'était plus Loulou ni Margot
Dont je serrais la taille fine…
It was no longer Loulou or Margot
whose narrow waist I held…

He scratches his head shyly. "That's it, eh. Not bad, not bad." Suddenly, he tosses back the sheets.

C'était la reine de l'Argentine
Et moi j'étais son hidalgo.
She was the queen of Argentina,
and I was her noble lord.

He begins to sing, quietly at first and then belting out the words, his raspy voice mingling with the cello's.

Ah! Ce que les femmes ont pu me plaire
Et ce que j'ai plu! J'étais si beau!
Oh! How I loved women,
and how they loved me! I was so handsome!

He sits up, animated now.

Faudrait pouvoir faire marche arrière
Comme on le fait pour danser le tango!
We should be able to go backwards,
like they do in the tango!

The music stops. "I had a great life," he says, "my youth was incredible. I had a blue motorbike, all blue. And I rode it to go out dancing! It was so good. There were some pretty girls, and I wasn't too bad myself." His eyes cloud over, lost in the distant past. "That's all over. We should be able to go back in time... But it was good, it was good. Oh, yes, it was. It's still good."

That good past, gone and buried, takes on the toothsome taste of the present.

Music is a living memory.
A light touch, a flash in the dark.
Old stories, the past
Becomes a surging, sensual present.
Time's steady slip,
The clock fallen silent,
The miracle of time reaches the heart beyond time.

Madame Azaro

"I feel like I'm really somebody!"

MADAME AZARO wants something high-pitched. "Fuck, you play really well, but it's all so dark."

She has advanced bronchial cancer as well as neuropsychiatric issues, partly due to brain metastasis.

Her life seems like something out of a film noir: a husband murdered and found in the trunk of his car, a daughter she hasn't heard from in twenty years, four brothers and sisters who drank and smoked and all of whom died of the same thing that's going to kill her too. She is a gossipy, hostile woman. She used to work as a lion tamer for the circus, before she was demoted, as she tells it, to cook's assistant. I meet Madame Azaro for the first time out on the terrace. She's sitting in her wheelchair, takes long, nervous drags of her cigarette, and starts coughing so hard she spits. "Being sick is so tedious."

When I play, she looks at me with her cloudy eyes, her lips swollen, her face gray. "I'd like some music that goes up, up, to the sun," she pleads hoarsely. "That's it, that's what I want. Can you do that? If I were up in the sun I could tell everybody exactly what I goddamn think."

The sound of the cello starts to rise, higher and higher. Madame Azaro is jubilant. When I'm with her I can feel that wavering that we all carry, between the inevitability of death and the desire to keep living. She's inspiring, this lion tamer, and I launch into wild improvisations, with frenetic tremolos that climb as high as the cello will go, and hysterical, whipped glissandi, harmonics bright as stars, calling for the raw light and pure air of the highest peaks. "Yeah! Bravo! Bravo," she shouts. "Thank you for the sunshine! Fucking hell... Up there in the light, I feel like I'm really somebody!"

Music is flight.
It breathes the mountain air.
In the struggle against the collapsing self,
Sound rises to the top of the sky.
It brings back identity,
Calls us to defy the fear of death,
And find ourselves in the bright midday sun.

Monsieur Fridman

"A balm upon my heart."

MONSIEUR FRIDMAN, seventy-six years old, has advanced prostate cancer. He is a man with fine features and an aristocratic manner and, in spite of his age, a full head of hair. He used to be a luxury clothing retailer, and has traveled all over the world. He has had six wives and many mistresses. The wives are at his bedside one after another almost without interruption. His days are complex to organize, and full of surprises.

As soon as I come into the room, he asks me without hesitation for Beethoven's "Ode to Joy." I am impressed by how closely he listens.

"I forgot that I'm in the hospital," he says at the end of the piece. "A beautiful woman came to romance me! I'll tell my wife." He blows me a kiss.

When I come back the following week, he has very specific musical requests. "First of all, the 'Nessun dorma' aria from the third act of Puccini's *Turandot*, if you please."

He is a cultivated man. He wields language with dexterity, and his comments are invariably pertinent. He talks about his taste for music, which goes back to childhood, and about his thirty-year subscription to the Théâtre des Champs-Élysées. He recounts juicy anecdotes about the famous artists he met on his many trips. Our encounters, to Verdi and Puccini arias, are lighthearted and even flirtatious. His company is delightful.

But two weeks later, I find a very sick man whose condition has deteriorated considerably. I play for him again. Lying on his bed, his face drawn, he watches the cello. When I finish the sarabande from Bach's Fifth Suite, Monsieur Fridman doesn't say a word. His lips quiver slightly. There's no more banter. He gives me a wan smile and, as I'm about to leave, he rolls up his sleeve without a word and shows me his Auschwitz number. I come back to the bed. He strokes the tattoo on his arm, and says, without looking at me, "In the face of the unspeakable and the unbearable, music ties us to the meaning of life. Thank you. It is a balm upon my heart."

Music is silence.
One by one, words fall
Along the way, useless baubles,
Empty shells.
Before mystery only silence remains
And the open wound that cannot be named.

Madame Bellec

"Long live Brittany!"

MADAME BELLEC doesn't want to live anymore. She has lung cancer, with liver metastases. She no longer communicates with anyone, not her only daughter or her caregivers, and she shows no interest in the Mozart arias I play for her. She remains silent during our first two sessions, staring straight ahead, her face closed. I learn from a nurse the following week that she was born in a little village near Quimper, in Brittany. During our third session, without saying anything, I launch into a traditional Breton ditty: "Vive la Bretagne." Madame Bellec jumps as if she's been pricked. Eyebrows raised, she meets my eyes, amazed.

"You recognize it?" She nods several times and stares at me intently. "More? Again?" "Yes, yes!" She speaks! "Yes, again."

Her eyes are lit up like hundred-watt bulbs. I play the same song for her. *Vive la Bretagne, vive les Bretons!* "I know it, know it. Again."

She's breathing fast. She lifts her head from the pillow— at least two inches. She's singing with me now, or mumbling, rather, but she's keeping the beat, shaking her head from side to side, her eyes bright. *"Vive la Bretagne, vive les Bretons!"* The song is quite bawdy, though I'd never really realized it before. She knows every word; now it's my turn to be amazed.

Quand il passe un aéroplane,
Tous les hommes lèvent les yeux,
Quand il passe une jolie femme,
Tous les hommes lèvent la queue.

She smiles. *When an airplane goes by, all the men raise their eyes. And when a pretty girl goes by, all the men raise their...* She hasn't smiled once since she's been on the unit. *"Vive la Bretagne,* madame musician, long live Brittany!"

When I come by the following week, she's gone. The nurses report that after our session she sang continuously until lights-out. She was smiling, too. Then she fell silent, and died two days later.

Music is a song from childhood.
It lets us be shaken,
Refreshed, it returns us to desire.
It waits at the edge of dry lips,
When everything else is gone.
A childhood song is a loving voice
That flows in the blood,
It illuminates the soul's final sigh
And gathers a whole life
In its delicate hands
Never asking a thing in return.

Monsieur Loiseau

"It's a way out."

MONSIEUR LOISEAU is forty-six. He's HIV-positive and has mela-
noma with brain metastases and hepatitis. He doesn't get any
visits. When I come into his room one November morning,
he welcomes me with a relieved smile and addresses me infor-
mally: "Play me something to calm me down, I had a horrible
night."

Cross-legged on his bed, he listens solemnly as I play
Gabriel Fauré's "After a Dream." "First, there's emotion," he
says, "then fragility. My hair is standing up on end." He
wraps his arms around his legs, folding in on himself. He's
so gaunt it's startling. As if talking to himself, he adds, "It's
like the music is giving me a way to make something burst out,
you know, not necessarily from within myself, but like some

outside force. As if the music wasn't meant for just one person, but many... It sounds nuts, but... a possible sharing." He turns his ravaged face to me: "Do you understand? Actually, I think it's my suffering that wants to come out. You're offering me a way to stop feeling tied up. It's a way out."

I play for him for a long time. "It gives some meaning to desiccated, dehumanized things," he says. Music runs through him like a current.

When I come back the following week, he's gotten much worse. He's lying on his bed, his body marbled, his face hidden behind an oxygen mask. He's been unconscious since the day before. His arms are folded over his chest. He looks like he's waiting. Yet when I play him the opening notes of the Fauré, his chest swells. The tempo of "After a Dream" matches his breathing, which gradually deepens. I have slipped into the rhythm of his breath; I have that privilege. He breathes with the song of my cello. There is only our breathing in the room, mysteriously attuned with the melody. A common pulse.

When I stop playing, I notice the goosebumps on his arms. After a dream.

It's our last exchange. He dies that same day, barely an hour after I leave his room.

Music is resonance.

It insinuates, echoes, connects.

Multiple sounds,

A multiplicity of emotions.

It reaches the person lying ill

In their lone, lived experience.

Music accepts difference

Fluently.

Goosebumps prove our presence in the world

Until the very end.

Life in its purest state at the threshold of the wide sky.

Madame Rameau

"It vibrates in my body and in my heart."

THE FIRST TIME I push open the door to her room, I am struck by Madame Rameau's beauty. Lying on her bed, her hands crossed, she seems very calm. She has lung cancer with brain, bone, and liver involvement. She is sixty-nine years old, elegant. She is wearing a purple headband and light eye makeup. Her skin is almost translucent. She turns to look at me, her eyes worried, but when she sees me she seems relieved: she's heard the cello through the wall, and she's been waiting, she wasn't sure it would get to her.

"I like music," she tells me, "but my husband is the real fan. It's too bad he's not here." Her face darkens.

Benjamin Britten's Cello Suite no. 3, with its ending like an Orthodox prayer, fills the room with dusky harmonics.

Madame Rameau closes her eyes and absorbs each sound fully: "That really resonates. It's strong. It vibrates in my body and in my heart. I never would have imagined that it could vibrate like that." I also play her Schubert's "Serenade" and Fauré's "Sicilienne." Madame Rameau beams at me. "I'm so sad that my husband isn't here. You'll have to come back."

The next week, he's the one who opens the door and welcomes me warmly, for a session that lasts over an hour, and which makes them both so happy. By request, I play the overture of Charpentier's *Te Deum*, excerpts of Mozart's Symphony no. 40, and a few opera arias. Music therapy becomes a full concert when he asks for Dvořák's Cello Concerto in B Minor. As I dive into the first movement, I think fleetingly of my teacher in Russia and the room where I had my lessons at the Moscow Conservatory. I play the cello solos and I belt out the orchestra parts. The performance is total chaos, and some might deem it a disaster, but I have an inkling that it's actually perfect.

In the infinite space of the universe we share, Moscow crumbles.

Moscow flickers on the horizon and sinks to the bottom of my fears.

The nurses stick their heads in the door and decide to come back later to give Madame Rameau her meds. The attendants do the same for lunch.

Madame Rameau's cheeks are pink and her eyes twinkle. She is completely changed by how happy her husband is, and she laughs at his almost childlike enthusiasm as he asks me with unabashed gluttony for another concerto, and another. Time stands still. They don't want me to leave. When I finally say goodbye, she turns to her husband and, pointing to her heart, says, "It soothes me. I'd forgotten that this was still alive, in here."

But when I come back the third time, Madame Rameau seems tired. Her husband, on the other hand, sees me and immediately places a new order: the slow movement of Schubert's Arpeggione Sonata. The patient's lips tremble imperceptibly. I see the furtive glances she gives him: she can feel how happy the cello music makes him. She would like to go on sharing it with him, but he's not looking at her. Within these four walls, the music's banal distraction feels like a growing tsunami. The situation is getting a little out of hand. I'm not in control anymore. Madame Rameau withdraws. I see her body shrinking, her hands knotted again. She is pale. She has been pushed aside, abandoned along the way. He will know how to be happy without her. She can see it in his glowing face. With all my strength, I focus on her, I look at her, smile at her. The threat of a whole being laid bare hovers dangerously as death draws near, and with it, the collapse of meaning. I know full well that her illness isn't my fault, nor will her death be; I'm not responsible for all the nuances of their lifelong relationship that escape me. I'm just passing through. But her deep despondency and her husband's obliviousness affect me too, and I carry it with me as I leave the room.

Music is light.
We aspire to remain whole and it subsists
In spite of the fragmented body.
The gaze of the other lets us fight against annihilation.
The other sees us, restores unity,
And shatters it into the void.
The same eyes.
The cello's vibrations drench the eyes in light.

Madame Adélaïde

"Thank you for allowing me to gladden my mother's heart."

TODAY IT'S THE PATIENT'S SON, a man in his fifties, who greets me when I come into the room. He seems a little frantic and doesn't look at me, and selects the most suitable chair for me—"not the wheelchair, not the armchair with armrests"— and the best location—"not too far from the light, not too close to the bathroom." His voice catches: "And especially as close as possible to my mother." Madame Adélaïde is ninety-one years old. She has terminal vulvar cancer, which has just been discovered. She's been on morphine for two days for the pain, and is drowsy and unresponsive.

I play Albinoni's Adagio, and her son, standing with his head against the wall, cries quietly. The piece ends, and he can't take his eyes off his mother. A long, full silence follows the music. It's always just the right amount of time, if you're willing to wait. His mother has always been surrounded by music, he tells me. Her husband, his father, was a water-colorist who listened to Bach while he painted. "It gets me right here," he explains, his hand over his heart, still not looking at me. "You have to play again. Bach."

So I go on, with several dances from Bach's Cello Suites, and Madame Adélaïde begins to breathe much more deeply, although she is unconscious; it's even more noticeable in the moments of silence between movements. "If she can hear," her son tells me, "it must be moving for her." He is calmer now. He's still staring at his mother, watching her chest rise and fall as she breathes, the sheet moving up and down. "Yes, she can hear," he says.

When I lift my bow to signal the end of the session, he looks me in the face for the first time. "Thank you," he says. "Thank you for allowing me to gladden my mother's heart. She's not suffering anymore now. You've given her a voice." He looks years younger.

The following week, a woman I haven't seen before stands in front of the half-open door. She's visibly angry and I can see by the look on her face that she is there to prevent me from coming in. As I walk away, a little nonchalantly, Madame Adélaïde's son flies out of the room like a whirlwind and catches up to me. In a jumble, he explains that his sister doesn't want music for their mother, but I have to ignore her. He begs me to come and play Bach. His sister rushes out after him and they argue in the hallway.

I watch the fight helplessly, an outburst of anger that I don't really understand. Just then, another sister arrives, with her husband and children, and tries in vain to calm them down. A little girl starts to cry. In an instant, I make up my mind, slip through the door, and settle quickly into the same chair as the last time—not the wheelchair, not the chair with armrests, not too far from the light, not too close to the bathroom. The silent stillness of the grandmother lying on her bed with her eyes closed is a strange contrast to the commotion outside.

Bach's aria. The cello's song cloaks the shouting in the hallway in velvet. The music seems to flow like a clear spring, like the sound of wings toward the sky. The song pivots slowly in the hospital-scented air. At that moment, I feel like this is the only possible answer to what has no answer. The shouts have fallen silent. One by one, the relatives enter the room. Only the rebellious sister remains at the door. Bach has grabbed them all by the sleeve and shaken them up a bit. Bach doesn't lecture them, he just offers a glimpse of an infinite grace, stronger than anger. Madame Adélaïde's breathing gradually expands; it's impressive. Perhaps the only way she has left to tell them that she's still here is her breath. Everyone has noticed the change in her breathing, and when the music dies down, the room seems lighter. It's amazing how sound can brighten things. I've seen it happen often. The son seems happy. The sister with the children is grateful: "It's beautiful, it's profound." The other sister is stock-still in the doorway, made of stone, but when I leave the room, the statue comes to life and follows me out. I know that I took a risk by playing, and I know it worked. She wants to talk to me. I stop, and turn toward her. "I didn't expect this," she says quickly, looking down at her shoes. "It held us together. It calmed us down."

Music is voice.

Death looms, strikes unspeakable fear.

The voice of the cello tries to loosen the stranglehold of silence.

It invites a community of emotions, sharing

In spite of the abject terror.

The chaotic heart,

Outbursts of rage.

The way of the cello fights as it does against the final betrayal.

A testament to the possibility of letting go.

It binds those who stand together

Around the bed of the dying.

Madame Cazeneuve

"Let me tell you a secret."

MADAME CAZENEUVE was a great actor, a senior member of the Comédie-Française. She is a handsome woman, with her hair pulled up into a high bun and rings sparkling on her fingers. She played all the great roles. The first time I met her at the Korian Jardins d'Alésia, she dismissed me, politely but firmly. I remember that she instantly went back to her book; the matter was closed.

Two years later, I come across her in palliative care at Sainte-Périne, an urgent transfer for terminal kidney and cardiac failure. When I come into her room, I find a frail figure curled up under the white sheets. I approach the bed gently and ask if she'd like to hear some music. She waves me over. Her face is unrecognizably thin, the bones poking through, though her eyes are still sharp, with the cutting edge of good kitchen knives.

"Let me tell you a secret," she whispers, beckoning me even closer. I lean over. "Get out of my room at once!" she shouts, so theatrically that I nearly drop my cello, my bow, my endpin stop, and my bag of scores.

Madame Cazeneuve—she was a character, right to the end.

Music is provocation.
It lends the strength to refuse,
The grace to say no,
Say it loud.
You have to hold on to life until the end
And never drop character
Especially if it's the last part you'll ever play.

Madame Bloch

"It will all come back."

MADAME BLOCH absolutely doesn't want any music. "I'm all alone, and if you play for me, I'm too afraid that—that it will all come back." She's been admitted to the unit for a chronic pain assessment. She is another Holocaust survivor, the only member of her family. She likes music, but no, sorry, she definitely does not want to hear the cello.

But a little later, as I'm leaving the room next to hers, I catch her with her ear to the door: when I push it open, the door smacks her in the head, quite hard. She shuffles away with her head down, caught off guard. The nurses tell me that she's been following me around like this since the morning, hiding behind every door, enjoying the cello as she chooses, and free to move away whenever the emotion becomes too intense. The music rouses some fundamental impulse in her, and she can't control it, so she's come up with a clever way to parcel out doses she can handle.

Music is danger.

Dark fears overwhelm the heart, the blood.

Some are so awful, they have no name.

Ancient, paralyzing fears.

Even sound-friends let them be.

They must not be disturbed.

They pretend to be sleeping.

They could wake up

Fangs out, kill us in a snap.

Madame Beauchamp

"It sounds like her voice."

WHEN I STEP INTO MADAME BEAUCHAMP'S ROOM for the first time, I'm wearing so much protective equipment that I look like an astronaut. Madame Beauchamp is sixty-two years old, with extremely aggressive multiresistant urinary and pulmonary bacterial infections. They've put her in isolation. I slip on the mask and gown before going in, though in the interest of playing in tune, I manage to negotiate with the nurse about the gloves.

Madame Beauchamp has a parkinsonian type multiple system atrophy, a neurodegenerative disease. Close up, I'm struck by how rigid her limbs and her neck are. She's lying across her bed like a desiccated tree, its trunk and branches gnarled by a violent storm. Her posture is so distorted she almost can't swallow at all. In any case, her jaw is clamped so tight it's impossible to even get her to open her mouth. Her skin is damaged, too: her left cheek is swollen, and she has sores on her collarbones and on her heels. Her head and neck look permanently crooked. She is completely paralyzed. Her eyes are wide open, tearless. They look like shiny stones. Yet she answers all the questions anyone asks, blinking once for yes, twice for no, while her body lies there, fragmented, broken.

The sparkle in her eyes reaches out to me, one living being to another. Instantly, we become friends. Despite the depth of her suffering as she nears the end of her life, she is completely alive. What draws me to her has very little to do with pity: there is something central, from the core or the heart, that pulls me in, even though I'm only passing through, only crossing her path for a time.

That impulse, ephemeral and blinding, requires all my hope and effort, every reason I have for living.

The cello? She blinks once. Blinks once again for classical music, and again, yes, something soft. One last blink for Bach's "Jesu, Joy of Man's Desiring."

When I begin to play the cantata, there is an immediate effect, like a tiny tremor. It's barely noticeable. Light as a butterfly's wings. Her eyelids move first. *Jesu, joy of man's desiring...* And then, all at once—I'm not expecting this at all—a flood bursts from her parched eyes. It surges forth, powerful as only water can be that has been held back for too long, gushing through a breached dam. It's terrifying. I keep playing, but I can feel the panic rising. What if I'm hurting her? Violent sobs contort her mouth and her whole face, even while her body remains completely immobile. Ignoring my momentary uncertainty, I decide to push through, all the way to the motet. *Jesu, joy of man's desiring…* She cries and cries, soaking her cheeks and her pillow. Then slowly, the tears abate, like the first rays of sun after a storm. I can only communicate with her through her eyes, but they're clear and bright, like a child's after hearing a story with a happy ending. I lean closer. "Did you like it?" Blink. "Would you like me to play again for you?" Blink. "Another cantata? Bach?" Blink.

I stay with her for a long time. She is calm now.

Bach's Cantata BWV 1 is called *Wie schön leuchtet der Morgenstern:* how beautifully the morning star shines.

Yes, she says again with her eyes.

Der Himmel lacht! Die Erde jubilieret! The heavens laugh, the earth exults; BWV 31.

She's beaming. She wants more, yes.

Liebster Gott, wenn werd ich sterben? Dearest God, when will I die? BWV 8.

The sound-friends, when they fade to stillness, leave behind silence, a quiet that quivers with the rustle of wings. Purveyance of joy.

Her husband is with us for all the subsequent sessions. Every Thursday, they wait for the astronaut-cellist to come play three cantatas among the many Bach wrote. "It's beautiful, it's melancholy," he says. "It's as rich as a human voice; it sounds like her voice." Madame Beauchamp cries often while the cello sings, but the early torrents have become rivulets. Her husband is overcome too, and strokes her hand. "It hits exactly where it should. My wife has come back to me."

The cello is a human voice, and Bach's is the voice of the heavens. I can see now that there is no difference between the two as they sing in unison over Madame Beauchamp's beautiful face.

She lived for five weeks after she stopped eating and drinking, in defiance of every single medical prediction.

Music is deliverance.
It calls forth tears we thought had gone dry.
It knows the moment
When the burden lifts.
It lets loose a salty spring, freely,
To go wherever it wants.

Monsieur Kahil

"Maghrebi rap."

MONSIEUR KAHIL is only twenty years old. He's pissed off: all his friends from school are on vacation, and he's stuck in bed. The cancer is everywhere in his body, and he's in constant pain, despite powerful, targeted drugs. He has an axillary tumor so massive it's chewed up his entire arm, like a monstrous poisonous mushroom. He doesn't want to look at himself in the mirror anymore, he tells the nurses. The pain wanders around inside him every second of the day, consummate and unbearable.

The first time we meet, he asks me to pass him his guitar, which is in a corner of the room, and he sings along with me to some Johnny Hallyday tunes. He knows a lot of chords, and he's a good musician. It seems to make him happy. "It makes me forget," he says.

The following week, he asks me for Maghrebi rap or metal—my choice. I must say, Monsieur Kahil, I don't know what to pick. I never learned much of either in Moscow! Rap isn't in my repertoire, and I'm honestly completely ignorant about metal, though I'm willing to try. "Next week, I promise."

The third week, his buddies are back, and eleven of them are crowded in the room around his bed. They pass him the guitar, but he's too tired to lift it, and the instrument just lies there across his body.

Hornet La Frappe, Ahmed Soultan, H-Kayne, DJ Key… My phone pumps out a rap beat, and I follow along; I'm committed, I'm all in, a Moroccan hip-hop cellist. Eleven smartphones film me as I play.

"You dig MBS?" You bet, Monsieur Kahil. Le Micro Brise le Silence is my brand-new bae, even though the love affair only started today.

Avec le micro on brise le silence,
On va plus loin que la violence.
You break silence with a mic,
Go beyond the violence.

I beat out the rhythm on the ancient varnished body of my cello, now become an African drum.

La rage m'élance, avec le micro je brise le silence
C'est pas une coïncidence si j'parle que d'violence.
Rage propels me, with the mic I break the silence
It's no coincidence if I'm talking only about violence.

I'm dancing in my chair as the young rappers huddle around the bed, the lights of their phones shaking like fireflies in the night.

Wǝʾlāš? Tǝnūḍ ǝṣ-ṣbāḥ,
bāš taʿrif wāš ṣra l-bārḥ fǝllēl
Why should you wake up in the morning
To find out what happened at night?

We are a sacred choir of thirteen.

Šḥāl men wāḥǝd māt? "Miʾa waʿišrūna qātil!"
Šḥāl tyettem min gellīl? Kull yōm ḥkāya wǝḥda.
How many people died? "A hundred twenty were slain!"
How many poor people were orphaned? The same story every day.

Monsieur Kahil is grooving with us, wiggling so much that his guitar almost slides off him. All his friends are laughing with him.

Je me rappelle avoir été enfant
Innocent, enfant innocent enfant
Innocent y a pas si longtemps
Je me rappelle avoir été enfant
Innocent, avoir vu le sang d'enfant
Innocent.

I remember being a child
Innocent, child innocent child
Innocent not so long ago
I remember being a child
Innocent, having seen the blood of a child
Innocent.

In room 207, the smartphones are swinging. Everyone's digging everything.

J'ai vu l'innocence figée en noir et blanc
Bout d'papier insignifiant, j'ai lu des
Hommages posthumes du noir sur blanc
Bout d'papier couleur rouge sang.
I saw innocence frozen in black and white
Insignificant piece of paper
I've read posthumous tributes in black and white
Blood-red piece of paper.

That monotone, syncopated voice.

Je me rappelle avoir été enfant
Innocent, enfant innocent enfant
Innocent y a pas si longtemps
Je me rappelle avoir été enfant
Innocent, avoir vu le sang d'enfant
Innocent.
I remember being a child
Innocent, child innocent child
Innocent not so long ago
I remember being a child
Innocent, having seen the blood of a child
Innocent.

The rhythm is twitchy, addictive, and the pressure builds up to a kaleidoscopic finale. I'm digging it.

Music is rhythm.
It makes an innocent child dance,
Angel in a blood-red mask.
Music tries to ward off pain, horror
For a few seconds.
Against injustice it is powerless,
Trapped in black and white.

Madame Ricci

"Madre, Madre... Come back!"

THE TWO YOUNG WOMEN on either side of the bed are shaking their mother. *"Madre... Madre!"*

Madame Ricci has been unresponsive since yesterday afternoon. Her daughters are begging her, in a frantic mixture of French, Italian, and Sicilian, not to leave them. *"Madre... Madre... Torna con noi! Madre... Torna!"* Come back, come back to us.

They shout, tugging at her. The patient, her eyes closed, her face emaciated, does not move. Their screams intensify when they see me enter with my cello. "Save her... Save her! Please!"

Last week we all sang "Quando me'n vo'" together, an aria from Puccini's *La Bohème*, which Madame Ricci loves more than anything. "*Suona Puccini, suona Puccini...* Please, bring her back to life." The daughters are hysterical.

"I can't bring anyone back to life, you know," I tell them, "but I can play Puccini's aria." They finally drop their mother's inert arms. I stand next to the bed and place the collection of Italian arias on my stand.

I play Puccini's "Quando me'n vo'."

Suddenly, Madame Ricci opens her eyes wide. Her eyes are so wide they fill the room; everything else disappears. Everyone is speechless. She stares at her daughters, and starts humming. "*Quando... quando...*" I shudder. The daughters weep with joy and clap their hands.

"*Madre! Madre!*"

Sometimes there are moments of fleeting light, bits of stars shooting across the day. A parcel of sky, like a tiny oasis.

Music is a dream.
A call to eternity, to the miraculous.
Its song of beauty is a defiance
Of death's shadow across our eyes.
It sets the world alight with joy.
And then bows down
Before the separation, too much to bear.

Madame Fontaine

"It must do you a world of good."

MADAME FONTAINE is seventy-eight years old. She has cancer and Alzheimer's. Her memory is only as old as the present moment, with a few wisps of a distant past as accurate as a Swiss clock. She likes Viennese waltzes. I play Johann Strauss's *Blue Danube*. Lying in bed, she begins to dance. She lifts the red hospital blanket delicately between her two fingers like the hem of a ball gown, and begins to swivel. "A beautiful dress is a must," she says conspiratorially, her eyes twinkling. "You look so happy," she tells me one day after a particularly twirly *Emperor Waltz*. I look at her, a little surprised. She looks both delighted and serious.

"It must be good for you, too. Oh, it must make you happy to play for me. Doesn't it?" I'm taken aback. But she goes on, in the same tone: "Doesn't your neck hurt, or your back? You look happy. It's nice… It must do you a world of good."

The joy is mine, too, truly. Good point, Madame Fontaine.

Music is joy.

It sparks the words of those who have lost them

Into blooming.

Elusive, it brings order to chaos,

To what seems like a confused mind.

The flow of joy from the heart

Explores transparent clouds.

The flow of joy from the sky

Wavers in feather-light spirals

To the heart, awakened with a start.

Madame Eleonora

"To dance the swan's death once more."

MADAME ELEONORA was a prima ballerina with the Paris Opera Ballet. She's waiting for me in room 409, and states her request without smiling. Pyotr Ilyich Tchaikovsky, *Swan Lake*. Then she closes her eyes. She listens, perfectly still.

"All my life I danced the Queen." She is staring at me gravely. "Thank you for allowing me to dance the swan's death once more."

Music is movement.

It carries,

Moves,

Raises up,

Takes us away.

It is the desire to fly.

It reveals the creative force of sound.

Invites the unfurling of invisible gestures.

Monsieur N'Daye

"What it feels like to want to live."

MONSIEUR N'DAYE is a former UNESCO official, a very cultivated man, originally from Mali. He's been admitted to the unit with metastatic prostate cancer. He asks me for Schubert's "Ave Maria." That's all he wants. He listens with his hands folded. "Thank you," he says. "That's a ten, as the kids say."

The sun floods the room. "It's more beautiful than a prayer. I'm going to be selfish and close my eyes to hoard it, to keep it all, stockpile everything sensitive. You put love in, and I get it all. My heart is full. You bring me something extraordinary. Extra… ordinary. It's like another world opening up, the only world that should bring people together."

Monsieur N'Daye is a wise man, like my friend Monsieur Koumba, the boxer whose room is down the hall. I'm still playing Vivaldi arias. He wants to talk: "I haven't received everything yet, and here's why..."

Beneath his oxygen mask, he speaks carefully, with long pauses between every sentence. "I haven't received everything yet because it will go on, later, tomorrow, the day after tomorrow, and until I die. An eternal fount. You've reminded me of what it feels like to want to live."

I'm touched by his words. It's the same thought Monsieur Koumba had as he described his emotion haloed with joy, like a nebulous body of water flowing in the shape of a river. I wish they could meet.

"You spread the love that flows within you," he says before I leave; "When love is at the core, that means there's life there. An eternal love. There's no need to be afraid. I feel full, I feel peaceful."

The next day, the two sages do meet: Monsieur N'Daye and Monsieur Koumba spend a whole afternoon together on the balcony overlooking the garden. For two days, they become great friends. Monsieur N'Daye dies a week later.

Music is an encounter.
It sparks a will to exist.
Pushes away discontent
To the far shore.
It celebrates,
Like a sparkling jewel,
Love at the core.
It escorts joy to the heart of the final feast.

My Mother

I can see my mother in the faces of those two wise friends. My mother was beautiful. Her face was so lovely that it always contained everything that is precious to me: it could reassure the whole world.

My mother was cheerful. She laughed easily; we had been laughing together since childhood, endless fits of laughter. She always had a ready smile.

My mother loved beauty. She loved it fiercely, passionately, like a lover. She valued it above all things and judged those who dismiss it harshly. Her idea of beauty had to do with the balance of the parts to the whole, in the Platonic sense. She had flawless taste, and could be uncompromising about it.

My mother never got tired or bored, and she wasn't afraid of solitude. She was courageous without having to try.

My mother liked order, and sought harmony in all things.

My mother knew French poetry, Shakespeare's plays, Italian primitive paintings, Greek art. She savored books more than food.

My mother was full of common sense yet completely removed from material concerns. She would grab the wrong coat or the wrong keys, get off at the wrong station. She had no idea how much bread cost. She delighted in everything, and was wildly amused by her own distraction.

My mother was an artist.

When she died, she left me and those I love an unwavering joy.

Death of a Friend

TWO MONTHS AFTER HE ARRIVES in palliative care, Monsieur Koumba is transferred to the geriatric ward two floors below. He won't come back to the unit, despite his and his son's repeated requests. I won't play for him again; the department head won't let me visit. To avoid favoritism and attachment, he says.

I run into Monsieur Koumba one afternoon under the big trees in the garden as I'm leaving the hospital, my cello on my back. He is sitting in his wheelchair in the sunshine with a nurse. He clasps my hands in his huge ones. "Claire, Claire, Claire…" He can't say anything else, and I can't say anything at all.

A few days later, he's found unconscious, trapped between his wheelchair and the toilet. He dies shortly afterward. The entire palliative care team is upset. I am too. I miss Monsieur Koumba. I would have loved to play Édith Piaf's "Non, je ne regrette rien" for him one more time.

There are some people who continue to shine on even in their absence, like the stillness after the music ends—present, alive, luminous.

Reunion

August 2018. Brittany.

"Strangers in the Night": Howard has always loved Sinatra. He sings along with the cello, sways softly, claps. His eyes are the same as they ever were—intensely attuned to the present, both smiling and a little sad. His laughter hasn't changed either—sudden, enormous, endless. He's happy. I've come back to play for him. I had promised him in the metro, then years passed and I forgot. For the past two years, since I found out that there was something wrong, I've been searching for him desperately.

I play for Howard outside, in the sun, on a terrace that overlooks the sea in the distance, in the bright Brittany summer. I'm going through Paul's favorite repertoire, from the cello-punching days at the center, the prelude to Bach's Fifth Cello Suite; and Dîlan, that incredible musician, her beloved allegro from the Shostakovich sonata; and Amélia too, the wild child, who would claw at everything, her slow movement from Schubert's Arpeggione Sonata; and finally David, his fabulous variations of transfigured intervals.

Howard's lifelong companion, who cares for him day and night, gently lays the baby violin from his clown show on his lap. This is the first time the tiny case has been opened since Buffo's last public appearance in January 2011.

Howard is ecstatic. He remembers everything, even if the words have left him and his ideas are muddled. Howard is a speaker, a writer, a scientist, yet he has never put much stock in words and ideas for their own sake. In his heart, he is first and foremost an artist and a healer. Above all, he loves sounds that speak, the spark of joy in people's eyes, and the undercurrent that thrums in every being.

The neurodegenerative disease that has been wearing away at him for several years has left the core of his heart intact.

Where the heart is, he is home. Fully present.

Epilogue

Schubert, Piano Trio no. 2 in E-flat Major, op. 100
Recapitulation

ONCE UPON A TIME, there was a woman named Madame Kessler, a great lady and a magnificent artist. She suffered a great deal, until one day, she was miraculously relieved of her pain by the andante movement of Schubert's Trio no. 2 played for her on the cello. Four years later, she was transferred to a palliative care unit.

I arrive early the morning of May 23, and I spot Madame Kessler's name on the patients' chart. I read the nurses' report in the change-of-shift notes.

21 May 2016: Madame Kessler, 95 years old, transfer from EHPAD Korian Jardins d'Alésia. Pain assessment.

Bath and procedures are painful. Patient moans and does not answer any questions. Premedication with morphine and midazolam.

22 May 2016: Patient continues to moan even in her sleep. Her limbs are tense. Pain eased somewhat at the end of the day, after two 5 mg morphine injections.

My heart is beating hard as I push open the door of room 403. I haven't seen Madame Kessler since I left the care home a year earlier. I walk up to her, clutching my cello. She's extremely thin, her skin translucent. I can almost see death hovering at her dry mouth. She opens her eyes and looks at me. A slight smile, riddled with fire. She still looks the same to me, that light blazing in her eyes. Schubert, Trio op. 100, andante. She can't move, but her breathing expands impressively under the taut sheets. Her body grows lighter. She seems to be made of only breath and light. Her deep blue eyes flash and follow my every move, so present that I doubt myself for a moment. She who has spoken and declaimed so much and for so long now cannot speak at all. She reminds me of a queen.

After playing, I lean toward her. "Thank you. You've given me so much." It's important to say thank you, and to have the grace to say it while there's still time. She blinks her eyes in answer. I have enough light to last me the rest of my life.

During the change-of-shift meeting, the on-duty nurse shares a strange phenomenon she witnessed that morning. While she was bathing Madame Kessler, she left the room to get a washcloth. When she came back, the patient's respiratory rate had increased to 42. She closed the door, and continued washing the patient. Her respiratory rate dropped to 30. When she opened the door again, it swelled back up immediately to 42. Door closed, 30. Door open, 42. The nurse realized that the open door allowed her to hear the cello singing in the room across the hall.

I see her again the following week, on May 30. She is even less responsive, but she still reacts to the cello. In fact, the cello is the only thing that seems to get a response out of her at all. Madame Kessler, who was admitted because she was in such pain, gradually cries out less. By early June, her pain is more or less under control. She relaxes, and stops moaning. Slowly, she begins to go. Like a boat that has been moored for a long time, one by one she releases the things that bind her and drifts out to the open ocean. She slips into a coma.

On June 6, during her final Schubert treatment, she already seems to be far away. Her splendid face looks like it's been chiseled from white marble, and it's bathed in an otherworldly light. Her eyes seem to be looking somewhere deep within. Her face is so naked, so exposed. I match my playing to her breath, busy as it is with the work of dying. One more time, for the last time, I play her the andante from Schubert's Trio. There are long pauses between breaths. I play a few measures with her warm exhale, a few in the cool absence of breath. It's like death is sitting on the edge of her bed, waiting for the end of the movement. But again life rushes into her body like the waves of the sea into a lonely reef, and a new breath comes to chase the last. Her whole life is held in her rib cage expanding. The astounding power of a life about to end. She is alongside the infinite.

"Goodbye, Madame Kessler."

That day, the file reads, "Schubert treatment with Claire. Incredible: The patient, drowsy and with limited responsiveness, sang."

On June 7, the day after the last song, after the Schubert treatment that began with her and which every week and for years has been taking people's pain away, Madame Kessler, a great lady and a magnificent artist, dies, alone, peacefully.

Undercurrent

My story isn't really done, but it stops here.

My singing cello, which treats those who have severe autism, long-term care home residents, patients with dementia, and people in great pain or in end-of-life care, is not pleasant entertainment, nor mere consolation, nor even a temporary alleviation.

The cello's vibrations touch, and fold, and traverse the failing body, coursing through it, invading it. The body itself vibrates and feels alive, it feels, it senses. It seems to resonate with the depth of existing.

Serious illness is an experience that dislocates us from ourselves. It attacks the body, and takes so many things from us—our ability to act, to do for ourselves. It leaves us bereft, strangers to ourselves, without a stable, familiar home.

Live music is transformative, a flash of life. It tears at the dormant heart, jump-starts it, proof of the philosopher Henri Bergson's observation, "Art would suffice then to show us that an extension of the faculties of perceiving is possible."

Music is a redeeming interruption that calls forth something from deep within us, unchanged and radiant, despite the fragmentation of illness, dementia, pain, and death. This core is common to all of us. It shines in us, between us, through us. It is subterranean, a constant undercurrent, the original mark. It holds life aloft. It is life.

Music seeps down underground, binding, miraculous.

A sense of trust.

The purveyance of joy.

Acknowledgments

For Howard Buten, the genius,
inspiring artist who showed me the way.

For Dr. Jean-Marie Gomas, a creative,
generous doctor, who helped pave it.

For Dr. Donatien Mallet, a true philosopher of care,
who helped guide me as I articulated what I saw along the way.

TRANSLATOR'S ACKNOWLEDGMENTS

As well as all those who help make books and translations,
including this one, my thanks specifically to Pablo Seib for
assistance with musical content, Dr. Claudia Finkelstein for
the medical terminology, Skye Nicholson, R.N., for the nursing
terminology, and Dr. Maria Pakkala for help with Arabic.

Notes

1   **Schubert, Piano Trio no. 2 in E-flat Major... Exposition:**
Classical sonata form, developed from 1750 onward, consists of
three main parts—the exposition, development, and recapitulation—which form a single movement. The three major moments of
Madame Kessler's story recounted here evoke the sonata structure.

6   **Slow, joyful:** Per M.-A. Charpentier, *Règles de composition*
(1690), a treatise that lists the expressive properties attributed
to the various major and minor musical modes or, in the
author's words, their "energy."

8   **I didn't even know these questions existed:** Joëlle Martineau
et al., "Electrophysical Evidence of Different Abilities to Form
Cross-Modal Associations in Children With Autistic Behavior,"
Electroencephalography and Clinical Neurophysiology 82, no. 1 (1992):
60–66.

8   **"They obviously have so much to teach us":** Howard Buten,
Ces enfants qui ne viennent pas d'une autre planète: Les Autistes
(Paris: Gallimard Jeunesse, 2001)

12   **"You have to look at them straight in the eye":** Howard Buten,
Il y a quelqu'un là-dedans: Des autismes (Paris: Odile Jacob,
2003), 46.

12   **there is someone in there:** The phrase refers to the title of
Buten's book, *Il y a quelqu'un là-dedans* ("There is someone in
there").

13   "his hoarse voice spitting out syllables": Howard Buten, *Through the Glass Wall: A Therapist's Lifelong Journey to Reach the Children of Autism* (New York: Bantam, 2004), 6.

13   *"Home,"* he emphasizes; "Where the heart is": Buten, *Through the Glass Wall,* 2.

15   Soft, tender: Per J.-P. Rameau, *Traité de l'harmonie réduite à ses principes naturels* (1722).

16   "Some days, I tell myself": Buten, *Il y a quelqu'un là-dedans,* 26.

18   "The doctor was always late, never absent": The descriptions of Georges Oppert cited in this chapter are taken from Jean Maheu's eulogy delivered at the funeral of Dr. Oppert, September 27, 1994, at the Jewish cemetery in Montparnasse.

21   Joyful, with gratitude: Rameau, *Traité de l'harmonie.*

23   "powerful desire for aloneness and sameness": Leo Kanner, "Autistic Disturbances of Affective Contact," *The Nervous Child* 2 (1943): 217–50. Case study.

23   "I believe they should be loved for what they are": Marie-France Bazzo, "Entrevues: Howard Buten," *Indicatif présent,* Radio-Canada, February 14, 2023.

24   "invisible wall": Buten, *Through the Glass Wall,* 22.

25   a Giuseppe Sammartini sonata: Giuseppe Baldassare Sammartini (1695–1750) was a late-Baroque Italian composer.

27   Sorrowful: Per Johann Mattheson, *Das neu-eröffnete Orchestre* (Hamburg, 1713).

28   "First, you have to earn their attention": Association des Paralysés de France, "Art thérapie, elle joue du violoncelle au chevet de patients," APF France handicap, September 14, 2009, dd84.blogs.apf.asso.fr/archive/2020/09/14/art-therapie-elle-joue-du-violoncelle-au-chevet-de-patients-129369.html.

29 "two-finger method": Buten, *Through the Glass Wall*, 58.

30 "I believe they have to be educated": Bazzo, "Entrevues: Howard Buten."

31 "Your gaze has to become a house": Buten, *Il y a quelqu'un là-dedans*, 144.

32 "Since no one really knows what to do": Quoted in Francis Marmande, "Autistes, artistes: À une lettre près," *Le Monde*, May 25, 2005, lemonde.fr/idees/article/2005/ 05/25/autistes-artistes-a-une-lettre-pres-par-francis-marmande_653729_3232.html. Original source unknown.

33 "I want to know what in the world": Buten, *Through the Glass Wall*, 6.

33 "A storyless journey through the hilly, heady land": Buten, *Through the Glass Wall*, 59.

45 her entire family moves in, fleeing Azerbaijan: The family was driven out of Azerbaijan in 1989 during the Nagorno-Karabakh war (1988–94) between Armenians in the disputed region of Artsakh/Nagorno-Karabakh and the Republic of Azerbaijan.

50 It smells delicious: Poems in this chapter written by residents.

52 "travellers to unimaginable lands": Oliver Sacks, *The Man Who Mistook His Wife for a Hat and Other Clinical Tales* (New York: Summit Books, 1985), ix.

53 though some may say they are losing their minds: The term "dementia" is from the Latin *demens*, to be out of one's mind.

61 a seamless *perpetuum mobile*: The Latin phrase means "perpetual motion"; musically, the term refers to a passage or piece with a continuous flow of notes, usually of insistently equal value and played at a rapid tempo.

64 **Albinoni, Adagio in G Minor:** The piece commonly known as "Albinoni's Adagio," which is attributed to the Baroque Venetian composer, was in fact largely written by the musicologist Remo Giazotto (1910–98), based allegedly on fragments he'd found of a trio sonata written by Albinoni.

69 **"artistic interventions":** Richard Forestier coined the term *opération artistique* (*Tout savoir sur l'art-thérapie*, Favre, 2012). According to Forestier, rather than the created product—i.e., the artistic work—an artistic intervention refers to the instance of creation itself and the communication established with the patient.

104 **different pain scales:** SBS: state behavioral scale; SVS: simple verbal scale.

104 **position changes during treatment:** Unnatural body positions may reveal unexpressed pain.

105 **"more courage to dare to be ourselves":** Marine Mignot, "Étude de l'influence de la musicothérapie sur le personnel infirmier lors d'un soin douloureux en unité de soins palliatifs" (Université de Nantes—UFR de médecine et techniques médicales, 2017–18).

115 **I am sometimes a researcher, digging deep—I identify the phenomenon, pointing to it—and sometimes I'm just a companion, walking, and feeling, alongside:** A reference to Donatien Mallet's book *La Médecine entre science et existence* (Paris: Vuibert/Espace éthique, 2007): "Le regard qui sent et le regard qui pointe," literally, the gaze that feels and the gaze that points.

131 **"Le Temps du tango":** Lyrics by Jean-Roger Caussimon. Recorded by Léo Ferré on the album *Encore du Léo Ferré*, Odeon, 1958.

165 **Bach's Cantata BWV 1:** The Bach-Werke-Verzeichnis (BWV) is the thematic catalogue of the works of Johann Sebastian Bach, compiled in 1950 by the German musicologist Wolfgang Schmieder.

169 *"Avec le micro on brise le silence… C'est pas une coïncidence si j'parle que d'violence"*: MBS, "Rap de Maghrébin," track 10 on *Le micro brise le silence*, Island Records/Universal, 1999.

170 *"Wəʿlāš? Tənūḍ əṣ-ṣbāḥ… Innocent"*: MBS, "Enfants innocents," track 12 on *Le micro brise le silence*, Island Records/Universal, 1999.

192 **Premedication with morphine and midazolam:** Midazolam is an anxiolytic drug used in palliative care to reduce anxiety or as a sedative when suffering cannot be relieved by other means.

195 **"Art would suffice then to show us":** Henri Bergson, *The Creative Mind: An Introduction to Metaphysics*, trans. Mabelle D. Andison (New York: Philosophical Library, 1946).

Bibliography

Abiven, Maurice. *Pour une mort plus humaine.* Issy-les-Moulineaux, France: Masson, 2004.

Bergson, Henri. *La Pensée et le mouvant.* Paris: Quadrige PUF, 1998.

———. *Matière et mémoire.* Paris: Quadrige PUF, 1982.

Bobin, Christian. *La Présence pure.* Paris: Gallimard, 2008.

———. *L'Homme-joie.* Paris: L'Iconoclaste, 2012.

———. *Un bruit de balançoire.* Paris: L'Iconoclaste, 2017.

Buten, Howard. *Ces enfants qui ne viennent pas d'une autre planète: Les Autistes.* Paris: Gallimard, 1995.

———. *Il y a quelqu'un là-dedans: Des autismes.* Paris: Odile Jacob, 2003.

———. *Through the Glass Wall: A Therapist's Lifelong Journey to Reach the Children of Autism.* New York: Bantam, 2004.

———. *When I Was Five I Killed Myself: A Novel.* New York: Overlook Press, 1981.

Châtel, Tanguy. *Vivants jusqu'à la mort: Accompagner la souffrance spirituelle en fin de vie.* Paris: Albin Michel, 2013.

de M'Uzan, Michel. *De l'art à la mort.* Paris: Gallimard, 1983.

Fiat, Éric. *Grandeurs et misères des hommes: Petit traité de dignité.* Paris: Larousse, 2010.

———. *La Pudeur*. Paris: Plon, 2016.

———. *Ode à la fatigue*. Paris: Éditions de l'Observatoire, 2018.

Forestier, Richard. *Tout savoir sur la musicothérapie*. Lausanne: Favre, 2012.

Gomas, Jean-Marie. *Soigner à domicile des malades en fin de vie*. Paris: Cerf, 1998.

Hirsch, Emmanuel. *Partir, l'accompagnement des mourants*, 2nd ed. Paris: Cerf, 1986.

Jacquemin, Dominique. *Éthique des soins palliatifs*. Malakoff, France: Dunod, 2004.

Jankélévitch, Vladimir. *La Mort*. Paris: Champs Flammarion, 1977.

Kübler-Ross, Elisabeth. *On Death and Dying*. New York: Simon & Schuster/Touchstone, 1969.

Lafay, Arlette. *La Douleur*. Paris: L'Harmattan, 1992.

Le Guay, Damien. *Le Fin Mot de la vie: Contre le mal mourir en France*. Paris: Cerf, 2014.

Levinas, Emmanuel. *Ethics and Infinity: Conversations With Philippe Nemo*. Translated by Richard Cohen. Pittsburgh: Duquesne University Press, 1985.

———. *Totality and Infinity: An Essay on Exteriority*. Translated by Alphonso Lingis. Pittsburgh: Duquesne University Press, 1969.

Mallet, Donatien. *La Médecine entre science et existence*. Paris: Vuibert/Espace éthique, 2007.

———. *Une clinique du corps*. Montpellier, France: Sauramps, 2020.

Richard, Marie-Sylvie. *Soigner la relation en fin de vie*. Malakoff, France: Dunod, 2004.

Ricot, Jacques. *Penser la fin de vie: L'Éthique au cœur d'un choix de société*. Prefaces by Jean Leonetti and Philippe Pozzo di Borgo. Rennes, France: Hygée Éditions, 2019.

Ruszniewski, Martine. *Face à la maladie grave*. Malakoff, France: Dunod, 2014.

Sacks, Oliver. *The Man Who Mistook His Wife for a Hat and Other Clinical Tales*. New York: Summit Books, 1985.

———. *Musicophilia: Tales of Music and the Brain*. New York: Vintage, 2007.

Saunders, Cicely. *Hospice and Palliative Care: An Interdisciplinary Approach*. London: Arnold, 1990.

Saunders, Cicely, Mary Baines, and Robert Dunlop. *Living With Dying: A Guide to Palliative Care*. Oxford: Oxford University Press, 1995.

Verspieren, Patrick. *Face à celui qui meurt*. Paris: Desclée de Brouwer, 1988.